ScrubTales™ Diagnostic Medical Sonographer

A Real-World Career Guide That Tells the Truth About Diagnostic Precision, Physical Endurance, and the Responsibility of Seeing What Others Cannot.

ScrubTales™ Series 1 — Core Clinical Careers

Mason Preddy

MASON MAISON
PUBLISHING™
REWRITING THE NARRATIVE
MASONMAISON.PUB

Copyright & Disclaimer

This book is intended for informational and educational purposes only. It is not intended to provide medical, legal, financial, or career-placement advice. Healthcare education requirements, certification standards, licensing rules, and employment practices vary by region and may change over time. Readers are encouraged to verify current requirements with accredited educational institutions, professional organizations, credentialing bodies, and regulatory agencies before making career decisions.

The author and publisher make no guarantees regarding employment outcomes, salary levels, certification eligibility, or career advancement. Individual results will vary based on education, performance, geographic location, labor market conditions, and personal circumstances.

Mason Maison™ Publishing

masonmaison.pub

Chapter 1
Welcome

Welcome — How to Use This Book

Choosing a healthcare career is not simply a decision about education or job availability. It is a decision about how you want to spend your days, how you want to use your strengths, and what kind of responsibility you want to carry over time. Diagnostic medical sonography is a profession built on precision, observation, and patient interaction—one that offers meaningful impact while demanding focus, stamina, and technical mastery.

This book is designed to help you see the career from the inside out. Rather than presenting only job descriptions and training requirements, you will experience real Day-in-the-Life narratives, practical hiring guidance, compensation realities, and structured reflection tools that help you evaluate whether the rhythm of this profession aligns with your personality, goals, and lifestyle.

You do not need to read this book from beginning to end in a single sitting. Many readers return to specific sections at different decision points—when exploring programs, preparing for interviews, evaluating job offers, or reassessing long-term direction. Treat this guide as a working reference, a decision companion, and a mirror for honest reflection.

Throughout the book, you will encounter tools designed to help you evaluate alignment, including the Fit Analyzer, the Role Fit Index, and reflection prompts intended to help you consider not only whether you *can* do the work, but whether you will want to do it for years in a way that supports both your professional growth and your life outside of work.

If this career fits you, the pages ahead will help you prepare intentionally. If another path ultimately fits better, the insights you gain here will still move you closer to a healthcare role that matches who you are.

Let's begin.

Chapter 2

Introduction to the SCRUBfits™ — Meet the SCRUBfits™

Before moving deeper into this career guide, you will begin meeting a set of characters who appear throughout the ScrubTales™ series: the **SCRUB*fits*™**. These characters are not mascots, personality labels, or stereotypes. They are alignment archetypes — visual and narrative reflections of how different personalities, strengths, and working styles show up across healthcare careers.

Healthcare is often presented as a simple question: *What job do you want?*

But the more important question is: *What kind of work environment, pace, responsibility level, and daily rhythm actually fits who you are?*

The **SCRUB*fits*™** exist to help you notice those differences.

As you move through Day-in-the-Life chapters, decision points, reflections, and specialty discussions, you will occasionally see a **SCRUB*fit*™** highlighted. When that happens, it is not telling you who you *should* be. Instead, it is offering a mirror — a way to recognize the types of people who tend to thrive in certain settings and why. Some readers will recognize themselves immediately in a particular archetype. Others will see parts of themselves reflected across several. Both reactions are useful.

For Diagnostic Medical Sonography, you will most often see characters who represent traits such as sustained focus, technical precision, pattern recognition, patient-centered calm, and comfort working in diagnostic uncertainty. These archetypes help illustrate an important truth: success in healthcare is not determined only by intelligence or training. It is shaped by the match between your wiring and the real daily demands of the role.

Later in the book, you will encounter the Mini **SCRUB*fit*™** Healthcare Career Assessment and the Role Fit reflection tools. Together with the **SCRUB*fits*™** characters, these tools are designed to help you evaluate not only whether you *can* do the work, but whether the work is likely to feel sustainable, meaningful, and aligned over time.

As you read, pay attention to which characters feel familiar, which environments energize you, and which daily rhythms feel natural rather than forced. That awareness is not a small detail — it is the foundation of long-term career alignment.

Chapter 3
Why This Career Matters

Why This Career Matters More Than Ever

Ultrasound used to be considered a “supporting role” in medicine — a tool that helped confirm what clinicians already suspected.

Not anymore.

Modern healthcare runs on **speed**, **accuracy**, **cost-effectiveness**, and **patient safety**. Ultrasound checks all four boxes. And with every passing year, the world relies more heavily on sonographers to deliver answers that shape everything from ER protocols to prenatal care to life-saving interventions.

But the rising importance of diagnostic medical sonography isn’t just a trend.

It’s a shift in **how medicine thinks**.

Let’s step into why

1. Ultrasound Is Now the Frontline Detector

In many hospitals, ultrasound is no longer the "follow-up" test — it's the **first test**.

Why?

Because it can reveal:

- free fluid
- gallbladder inflammation
- appendiceal swelling
- kidney obstruction
- fetal viability
- DVTs
- ectopic pregnancies
- cardiac function
- vascular compromise

—all **faster** and **safer** than alternatives.

What used to take hours, sonographers now find in minutes.

Medicine is learning what sonographers have always known:

Sound sees the truth quickly.

2. The World Is Moving Toward Noninvasive Everything

We're entering a healthcare era where:

- the fewer incisions, the better

- the less radiation, the better
- the less cost, the better
- the earlier the diagnosis, the better

Ultrasound sits at the perfect intersection of all four.

It's the imaging modality that says:

"Let me show you what's wrong without cutting, burning, injecting, or radiating you."

That makes sonographers invaluable — not eventually, but **right now**.

3. Sonographers Are Becoming the Gatekeepers of Care

Your images decide:

- Is this patient admitted or discharged?
- Is this pregnancy viable or not?
- Does this patient need emergency surgery?
- Can this clot kill them?
- Do we need a CT or MRI next, or is ultrasound enough?
- Is this a minor problem or a major one?

The physician may order the test.

But **what you see becomes the path forward.**

That makes the sonographer's presence indispensable.

4. We're Facing a Global Shortage of Skilled Sonographers

This career is exploding — not slowly, not quietly, but urgently.

Hospitals can't hire fast enough.

Outpatient centers are expanding.

OB offices are booked months out.

Vascular labs need coverage yesterday.

Emergency departments are leaning heavily on ultrasound during triage.

Why?

Because demand has skyrocketed in:

- high-risk pregnancies
- cardiac disease
- stroke risk
- trauma care
- cancer detection
- bedside imaging
- rural healthcare

And because sonography is precise, immediate, and cost-effective, it is becoming the backbone of patient flow.

The world is short on people who can read the body through sound.

If you can, you're gold.

5. Ultrasound Is Becoming the ER's Third Language

In trauma bays across the country, you'll see three things:

- people shouting
- monitors beeping
- ultrasound screens glowing

Sonographers are equal parts calm and crucial.

The trauma team waits for a sentence that comes only from you:

"Yes, there's free fluid."

or

"No, we're clear."

One sentence changes the entire room.

This is what "vital" looks like in real time.

6. Technology Is Getting Better — But It Still Needs Humans

AI will evolve.

Ultrasound machines will get smarter.

Screens will get sharper.

But there is one thing AI cannot replace:

The sonographer's intuition.

The subtle tilt of the probe.

The precise adjustment of pressure.

The choice to scan one more angle.

The ability to read the patient's body language.

The decision to hunt for what "feels off."

Ultrasound is not plug-and-play.

It is technique, troubleshooting, finesse, and emotional intelligence —

all at once.

Machines don't interpret shadows.

Humans do.

7. Patients Trust Sonographers Instantly

Maybe it's the quiet room.

Maybe it's the soft gel.

Maybe it's the way you stand close, guiding breath and movement.

Maybe it's the intimacy of the work.

But something happens between patients and sonographers that doesn't happen anywhere else in healthcare:

People tell sonographers the truth.

They whisper fears.

They confess symptoms.

They admit what they didn't tell the doctor.

A sonographer becomes:

- a safe space

- a soft landing
- a steadying presence
- a silent witness

That trust is not small.

That trust is not accidental.

That trust is why the career matters.

8. Ultrasound Is the Future of Global Medicine

In remote villages, in underserved communities, in mobile clinics, in disaster zones —

ultrasound is often the only imaging available.

It can be carried, powered by battery, and used in environments where no CT or MRI could ever go.

In the future, more lives around the world will be diagnosed, reassured, treated, or saved by the hands of a sonographer than any other imaging professional.

That makes this career not just meaningful —

but globally essential.

The Bottom Line

This career matters more than ever because:

- it saves lives
- it provides clarity
- it reduces cost
- it preserves safety

- it works anywhere
- it works on anyone
- it works in real time

And behind the technology is the human being holding the transducer —

the one who sees what no one else sees.

That's you.

That's this career.

That's why we're here.

Chapter 4

Role in Modern Medicine

A Sonographer's Role in Modern Medicine

If you walked into a hospital and followed the path of a single patient—from the moment they arrive to the moment they leave—you'd see one constant woven through their journey, often quietly:

the sonographer.

Not always first, not always last, but always precisely when it matters most.

Sonographers stand at the intersection of diagnosis, direction, and decision-making, translating the body's secrets into answers that clinicians rely on. Their work is not linear; it is a web—touching almost every department, every specialty, every stage of care.

Let's step through the hospital the way a sonographer does:

room by room, hallway by hallway, story by story.

In the Emergency Department:

The First Calm in the Chaos

The ED runs on adrenaline, speed, and triage. People pour through the doors unsure of what's happening inside their own bodies. Nurses assess. Physicians prioritize. But when the words "ultrasound is coming" echo through the room, the chaos shifts.

The sonographer arrives with quiet intensity, rolling in the machine like a truth detector.

Trauma team waiting.

Surgeon watching the monitor.

Charge nurse hovering with meds.

The sonographer's job in that moment is absolute:

Find the answer.

Find it fast.

Find it clearly.

One sweep can change everything.

In Labor & Delivery:

The Keeper of Heartbeats**

Down the hall, the world feels softer—but no less urgent.

Here, sonographers influence:

- induction decisions
- emergency C-section calls

• fetal monitoring changes

• NICU preparedness

• patient reassurance during high-risk pregnancies

When a mother comes in terrified because she hasn't felt movement, it is the sonographer who dims the lights, applies the gel, and seeks out the flicker of life.

In these rooms, ultrasound is more than imaging.

It is hope made visible.

In General Radiology:

The Detective's Office**

This is where the mysteries land.

Abdominal pain.

Liver lesions.

Kidney concerns.

Unexplained swelling.

Masses no one can quite identify.

Sonographers move methodically, patiently, scanning millimeter by millimeter until the truth sharpens into focus.

They don't just "take pictures."

They **create** images that must be:

• diagnostically useful

• anatomically correct

- labeled with precision
- captured from multiple angles
- clear enough for the radiologist to trust

A misangled image can misguide a diagnosis.

A missed structure can change treatment.

A single shadow can shift the story.

The responsibility is enormous—but aligned sonographers rise to it with quiet pride.

In Vascular Labs:

The Guardians of Circulation**

Vascular sonographers are the ones who catch:

- blood clots
- arterial blockages
- aneurysms
- compromised flow
- post-operative changes
- stroke risk

The room is quiet.

The patient is still.

The sonographer compresses, measures, listens, analyzes, and documents.

Vascular ultrasound is its own language—one of rhythm, pressure, and subtle changes.

In these labs, sonographers are not just testers.

They are **lifesavers** disguised in scrubs.

In Cardiology:

The Heart Interpreters**

Cardiac sonographers see the body's most vital engine in motion. They watch valves open and close, chambers fill and empty, muscle walls thicken and slacken.

They assess:

- heart failure
- congenital defects
- fluid around the heart
- valve damage
- structural abnormalities
- post-surgical function

The cardiologist trusts the sonographer to provide windows into a beating world the naked eye will never see.

Their images become the blueprint of treatment.

In Breast Centers:

The Quiet Courage Rooms**

Breast ultrasound requires both precision and deep empathy.

A mass found on mammogram.

A lump someone felt in the shower.

A follow-up after biopsy.

These rooms are sacred.

Time slows here.

Fear expands.

Sonographers know they may be seeing something that will change a woman's life. Their voice—steady, warm, gentle—often carries the patient through the hardest minutes of her week, her month, or her year.

The machine hums.

The patient breathes.

The truth emerges.

And the sonographer holds the weight with grace.

In Surgical & Interventional Suites:

The Real-Time Navigators**

In the OR, the sonographer becomes the surgeon's second sight.

They guide:

- biopsies
- drain placements
- surgical navigation
- intraoperative imaging
- vascular access

Their hands must be steady.

Their timing must be exact.

Their confidence must be unshakeable.

Every angle matters.

Every shadow matters.

Every second matters.

In Outpatient Clinics:

The Continuity of Care**

Here, sonographers see patients repeatedly—building relationships that span:

- pregnancies
- chronic conditions
- long-term monitoring
- pre- and post-treatment imaging
- wellness evaluations

These rooms are filled with:

- familiarity
- conversation
- education
- reassurance

Sonographers often become the most consistent face in a patient's diagnostic journey.

In Rural & Mobile Medicine:

The Lifeline on Wheels**

Where CT and MRI can't go, where specialists are days away, where small clinics do their best with limited resources—sonographers bridge the gap.

They bring:

- early detection
- triage
- pregnancy care
- trauma evaluation
- chronic disease monitoring

In many parts of the world, the sonographer *is* the imaging department.

Their presence changes outcomes.

Their skills change lives.

The Truth at the Center of Every Department

Wherever the sonographer goes—ED, L&D, radiology, vascular, cardiology, outpatient, rural, surgical—one truth remains:

Their images shape the next step in a patient's story.

It is not exaggeration to say:

Modern medicine cannot function without sonographers.

Not well.

Not safely.

Not quickly.

Not compassionately.

And that is why sonographers don't just hold a role.

They hold a place.

A presence.

A purpose.

A critical thread woven through every care pathway.

Chapter 5

Myths and Truths about Sonographers

Myths About Sonographers (and the Truths Beneath Them)

Every healthcare career collects myths — half-truths whispered in waiting rooms, assumptions repeated in hallways, and ideas shaped more by what people *see* than what actually happens behind the scenes.

Sonography is no different.

In fact, diagnostic medical sonographers might be one of the most misunderstood professions in the entire hospital ecosystem. People think they know what sonographers do because they've *seen* an ultrasound. The dim room. The gel. The grainy picture on a screen.

It all looks simple.

Predictable.

Soft.

But myths — especially comforting ones — are rarely accurate.

This chapter pulls back the curtain on the illusions that surround the role and reveals the truth that lives beneath.

Because understanding this career means understanding not just what it is...

but what it is *not*.

****MYTH #1**

“Sonographers just push buttons and take pictures.”**

This is one of the most persistent misconceptions in the field.

Photography is capturing.

Sonography is **creating**.

The sonographer controls:

- angles
- depth
- pressure
- Doppler
- windows
- timing
- breath holds
- patient positioning
- anatomical correlation

The image is not “there” waiting to be photographed.

It is built, second by second, through technique.

If the sonographer doesn't find it, it's not found.

TRUTH: Sonographers are not picture-takers — they are real-time anatomists guiding the machine to reveal the unseen.

****MYTH #2**

"They can see everything."**

No imaging modality is perfect.

Ultrasound can be blocked by:

- bone
- bowel gas
- obesity
- surgical dressings
- air in tissues
- patient inability to position
- pain that prevents compression

Patients often say:

"But can't you just look? Can't the machine find it?"

But the machine only knows what the **sonographer** can coax into view.

TRUTH: Sonographers don't see "everything."

They see what's possible through physics, anatomy, and skill — and they fight for the best window every time.

**MYTH #3

"Sonographers only do baby scans."**

Ask any sonographer what the public thinks they do, and they'll laugh.

Mention "ultrasound," and most people picture:

- gender reveals
- cute sonogram printouts
- gel on a pregnant belly

But OB is only **one** branch.

Sonographers also evaluate:

- trauma
- gallbladders
- kidneys
- livers
- spleens
- blood clots
- aneurysms
- breast masses
- appendicitis
- cardiac function
- thyroid nodules
- unexplained swelling

• post-op complications

Ultrasound touches almost every organ system.

TRUTH: Sonographers aren't "baby people."

They're full-body detectives.

****MYTH #4**

"They can tell you the results."**

Patients often ask:

"What do you see?"

"Is everything okay?"

"Do I need surgery?"

"Is there a heartbeat?"

"Does it look bad?"

"Is it cancer?"

Sonographers know more than they'll ever be allowed to say.

They can't diagnose.

They can't interpret.

They can't hint.

They can't reassure falsely.

They can't reveal prematurely.

This creates one of the most emotionally complex parts of the job:

knowing the truth without being allowed to speak it.

TRUTH: Sonographers carry a thousand unsaid sentences every week — and they honor the boundary because patient safety depends on it.

****MYTH #5**

"The job is easy and relaxing."**

Soft music. Dim lights. Warm gel.

People think sonographers live in a spa.

But the reality includes:

- 12-hour shifts
- shoulder strain
- tendonitis
- scanning patients who cannot move
- imaging in trauma bays
- miscarriage confirmations
- elderly patients crying in fear
- children who won't hold still
- stroke codes
- surgical deadlines
- critical findings
- emotional heaviness
- nonstop add-ons

This is **physical** work.

This is **emotional** work.

This is **cognitive** work.

TRUTH: Sonography is not a relaxing job — it is a physically demanding, mentally intense, emotionally layered profession requiring endurance and precision.

****MYTH #6**

“Ultrasound can’t diagnose anything serious.”**

People assume ultrasound is the “soft” imaging.

But sonographers diagnose:

- ectopic pregnancies
- deep vein thrombosis
- gallbladder infections
- ovarian torsion
- appendicitis
- liver disease
- heart failure
- fetal abnormalities
- abdominal bleeds
- aneurysms

Ultrasound may look gentle, but its findings are some of the most life-changing.

TRUTH: Ultrasound is often the *first* line of detection for conditions that require immediate intervention.

**MYTH #7

"AI will replace sonographers."**

Here's what AI can do:

• detect patterns

• measure structures

• assist with documentation

• standardize scan protocols

Here's what AI **cannot** do:

• reposition a patient in pain

• coax a terrified child into stillness

• interpret emotional cues

• manage trauma bay tension

• decide where to look when something feels off

• find an image when the anatomy is hiding

• deliver comfort during devastating news

Ultrasound is one of the most human-dependent imaging modalities.

TRUTH: AI will support sonographers — not replace them.

**MYTH #8

"Anyone can do it after a short training."**

Sonography programs are intensive.

Clinical rotations are rigorous.

Mastery takes **years**, not months.

The job is not:

- scanning routines
- pushing presets
- memorizing anatomy charts

It is:

- interpreting shadows
- chasing whispers
- sensing abnormalities
- adjusting technique
- predicting angles
- managing pressure
- making judgment calls

And doing all of it **in real time**.

TRUTH: Sonography is a profession that requires training, endurance, intuition, anatomical fluency, and emotional intelligence.

****MYTH #9**

“Sonographers are support staff.”**

No.

Sonographers are:

- diagnosticians

• collaborators

• clinical anchors

• frontline responders

• navigators of uncertainty

The healthcare system depends on their clarity, competence, and steadiness.

TRUTH: Sonographers are clinical decision-makers — silently shaping the direction of care with every sweep of the probe.

**MYTH #10

"Ultrasound is simple."**

People say this because they've never held the probe.

Nothing about this work is simple.

It is an art.

It is a science.

It is a discipline.

It is an emotional undertaking.

And yet sonographers make it look effortless — because excellence always looks like magic to those who haven't practiced it.

TRUTH: Ultrasound is one of the most deceptively complex crafts in all of medicine. And sonographers are the artisans who master it.

Chapter 6

Heart of the Pulse

The Heart of the Precision Pulse

Every SCRUBfit™ category has its own rhythm.

Some careers move at the speed of adrenaline.

Some move at the pace of long, unfolding stories.

Some careers live in the world of numbers, others in the world of words.

The Precision Pulse lives somewhere else entirely.

It lives in the space between silence and sound, between shadow and clarity, between "something feels wrong" and "here is where, here is why."

Diagnostic Medical Sonographers are the core members of this category. If you stripped away the job titles and left only the way they think, feel, and move through the world, you'd still recognize them instantly.

They are the ones who can stand in a quiet room and change the course of someone's life without raising their voice.

They don't need a microphone.

They have a probe.

What Defines the Precision Pulse

The Precision Pulse is built on a handful of deep traits that show up again and again in sonographers who love their work:

They notice patterns.

They tolerate tension.

They move gently but think sharply.

They can be fully present for ten minutes, then reset and do it again.

Some of the core qualities:

- A steady, observant mind
- A high tolerance for ambiguity
- Respect for small details
- The ability to be kind without collapsing
- Curiosity about how things work beneath the surface

People in this category are rarely the loudest voices in a department.

But they're often the ones everyone turns to when something doesn't make sense.

The Precision Pulse Way of Seeing

The Precision Pulse doesn't just look at a screen.

They look at everything:

- How the patient is breathing
- How their story doesn't quite match their symptoms
- How a vessel compresses, then suddenly doesn't
- How fluid pools where it shouldn't
- How a fetal heartbeat sounds just a little too fast or too slow

They're always collecting data—visual, emotional, contextual—and quietly weaving it into a picture that others can act on.

This is not the kind of work you can do on autopilot.

It demands both attention and intention.

The Emotional Signature of the Precision Pulse

There is a particular emotional flavor to this category.

They are:

- Calm but not cold
- Empathic but not overwhelmed
- Serious about the work but gentle with the person in front of them

They know how to stay with someone in a hard moment without promising what they can't control. They know how to be present without taking every story home like a wound.

Over time, many sonographers in this category develop their own quiet rituals to stay grounded:

- pausing for a breath before walking into a difficult scan
- saying a silent intention before a trauma case
- writing down moments of joy to balance the grief
- sharing hard cases with trusted colleagues instead of carrying them alone

The heart of the Precision Pulse is not made of stone.

It's made of something far stronger:

a softness that has learned how to stay.

The Precision Pulse in the Wider Healthcare World

In the larger ecosystem of healthcare, the Precision Pulse often functions as:

- the tie-breaker when a diagnosis is unclear
- the calm anchor when emotions run high
- the quiet consultant when doctors need more information
- the early warning system when something dangerous is just beginning to appear

Their influence is often invisible to patients but unmistakable to teams.

A sonographer's findings can:

- confirm a hunch
- overturn an assumption

- escalate a concern
- prevent an unnecessary procedure
- prompt urgent intervention

They don't write orders.

They don't prescribe.

They don't operate.

But the work they do often decides which orders get written, which prescriptions get chosen, and which operations happen at all.

Where the Precision Pulse Overlaps with Other Categories

You'll see Precision Pulse energy in other careers too:

- the pharmacist who catches dangerous interactions before anyone else
- the ICU nurse who notices subtle changes and calls the team early
- the lab professional who triple-checks an unusual result
- the respiratory therapist who hears a change in breath sounds before the monitor alarms

What they all share is this:

They don't just do tasks.

They interpret the story the body is trying to tell.

For diagnostic medical sonographers, that story arrives in waves of gray and motion, sound and silence.

Why This Category Needs You

If you are someone who:

- notices when things are slightly "off"
- can stay calm when other people get loud
- likes solving puzzles without needing applause
- cares deeply but doesn't need to be the center of attention
- finds yourself quietly anchoring others in stressful situations

...then the heart of the Precision Pulse may already be beating in you.

You are exactly the kind of person this category was built for.

And sonography might not just be a good job for you.

It might feel like home.

From here, we'll start moving toward the lived experience—the days, the scans, the real people behind the role.

Next up, we step fully into story.

When you're ready:

Chapter 7

The Toll Booth

The Emotional, Cognitive, and Lifestyle Cost of Diagnostic Medical Sonography

Every healthcare career asks for something in return. Some roles demand physical endurance. Others demand emotional resilience, rapid decision-making, or constant multitasking under pressure. Diagnostic medical sonography asks for a quieter but equally real combination: sustained concentration, physical repetition, emotional presence with patients, and the responsibility of capturing images that may determine the course of someone's care.

The physical toll is often the first reality new professionals notice. Sonographers spend long hours standing, leaning, reaching, and maintaining steady probe pressure while adjusting equipment and positioning patients. Over time, repetitive shoulder, wrist, neck, and back strain can accumulate, particularly in high-volume imaging environments. Proper ergonomics, stretching, and workload awareness are not optional habits in this field; they are career-length protection strategies.

The cognitive toll is more subtle but just as important. Sonographers must remain intensely focused for extended periods while interpreting real-time anatomical images, adjusting techniques on the fly, and ensuring that no critical structure is missed. Even routine studies require continuous attention to detail, while complex cases demand rapid problem-solving and close collaboration with radiologists and physicians. The responsibility of knowing that incomplete or unclear imaging can delay diagnosis adds a level of quiet pressure that many outsiders never see.

There is also an emotional dimension. Sonographers often meet patients during moments of uncertainty—pregnancy concerns, unexplained symptoms, suspected disease, or emergency evaluations. Patients may ask questions you cannot answer or look to you for reassurance while you must maintain professional neutrality until physicians interpret the results. Learning how to remain compassionate without carrying every emotional moment home is a skill that develops over time, but it is part of the work.

Lifestyle costs vary by setting. Hospital-based sonographers may work evenings, weekends, or on-call rotations, while outpatient imaging centers may offer more predictable schedules but higher daily volume. Some environments emphasize speed and throughput; others emphasize specialty expertise and longer studies. Understanding how different work settings shape daily pace, stress levels, and recovery time is essential when evaluating long-term fit.

None of these costs are reasons to avoid the profession. They are realities to understand clearly before entering it. Many sonographers find deep satisfaction in the blend of patient interaction, technical mastery, and diagnostic contribution the role provides. The key is recognizing whether the daily rhythm—the posture demands, the concentration required, the emotional exposure, and the workflow expectations—aligns with how you function best over years, not just during training.

Alignment does not mean choosing the easiest path. It means choosing the path whose demands you can sustain without quietly wearing yourself down.

Chapter 8
The Real Work

Inside the Rhythm, Reality, and Identity of This Career

Most people think sonographers "do ultrasounds." They imagine you simply press a probe to a belly and images appear like magic. But the reality of this profession is more complex, more cognitive, more emotionally textured, and far more important than the public ever understands. Diagnostic Medical Sonographers are not machine operators — they are anatomical interpreters, clinical investigators, patient communicators, and critical members of the diagnostic chain.

This chapter takes you deeper than job descriptions or school brochures. It shows you the *living* layers of the profession — the physical demands, emotional moments, sensory environment, identity traits, stress points, satisfiers, and the invisible work that makes sonographers the backbone of modern diagnostics.

The Cognitive Work: Seeing What Others Can't

A sonographer is, above all else, a visual detective. The work requires:

- pattern recognition
- anatomical mapping
- spatial reasoning
- hand–eye coordination
- real-time decision-making
- emotional awareness
- technical precision
- the ability to understand what *should* be there vs. what *is* there

The average person never considers what it means to turn grayscale noise into an actionable finding. To be a sonographer is to train your brain to see subtle abnormalities in shadows, angles, and echoes that would look indistinguishable to almost anyone else.

A tiny echogenic focus.

A missing flow pattern.

A shape that doesn't match the norm.

A flicker of motion that should be smooth but isn't.

These are not "images." They are **clues** — and the sonographer is the one responsible for capturing them with accuracy, clarity, and intention. A physician may read the report, but the sonographer is the person who *built* the report's foundation.

Without a perfect image, there is no perfect diagnosis.

And that weight — that combination of skill and responsibility — becomes part of the sonographer's identity.

The Emotional Work: Patients Arrive With Stories, Not Just Symptoms

Every patient who walks into a sonography room brings a story, even if they don't speak it.

Some bring fear.

Some bring hope.

Some bring grief they haven't named yet.

Some bring denial.

Some bring curiosity.

And some bring the quiet expectation that you're about to change their life.

Sonographers witness the entire emotional spectrum of healthcare:

- the joy of a first heartbeat
- the tremble of a parent worried about a fetus
- the silence after discovering no cardiac activity
- the anxiety of a patient awaiting cancer follow-up
- the relief when a long-feared pathology is absent
- the gratitude after a painful procedure is ruled out

In this room, the lighting is soft, the sound minimal, the environment intimate. Many patients disclose things here they haven't told anyone else. They feel safe in the quiet.

A sonographer must balance professionalism with compassion—reassuring without overstepping, calm without detachment, supportive without promising results they cannot give.

This emotional agility becomes one of the profession's most underrated strengths.

The Physical Work: The Ergonomics You Never Hear About

The physical demands of sonography are real — and relentless.

You hold a transducer for hours at a time.

You freeze, rotate, lift, angle, and torque your wrist in micro-variations that compound over time.

You press through adipose tissue.

You adjust position based on patient limitations, pain, or mobility.

You lean over beds.

You balance your body to compensate for stretcher height or ICU constraints.

You scan in the OR, ED, cath lab, NICU, or bedside — each setting with different ergonomic challenges.

The profession asks for:

- shoulder strength

- wrist endurance
- core stability
- posture mindfulness
- ergonomic awareness

When sonographers say, "We feel it in our bodies," it's not an exaggeration — it's the truth.

Physical longevity is tied to alignment, environment, and technique.

The better matched a sonographer is to their specialty, the longer they can thrive

The Sensory Environment: The Soundless Pulse of the Room

Sonography rooms are different from any other healthcare spaces. They are:

Quiet.

Dim.

Focused.

Private.

Emotionally charged.

The lighting lowers your heart rate.

The silence heightens concentration.

The isolation amplifies both connection and tension.

Some people find this environment soothing—almost meditative.

Others find it draining, lonely, or emotionally heavy.

Your instinctive response to this environment is one of the biggest indicators of **alignment**.

Some personalities crave the calm. Others need more buzz, noise, teamwork, or stimulation.

This is why the **SCRUB*fit*™ Healthcare Career Assessment** is so critical. It helps you identify the emotional and sensory environments in which you naturally thrive.

The Identity Work: Who Thrives in Sonography

Certain personality traits make this career feel like home.

Sonographers tend to be:

- calm
- patient
- curious
- observant
- gentle
- investigative
- methodical
- detail-oriented
- adaptable
- compassionate

• steady

They are comfortable holding emotional space for patients while also making technical decisions moment by moment. They like seeing the "why" behind symptoms. They feel satisfaction when they find the answer that explains a patient's pain or concern.

They are not spotlight-seekers.

They don't crave chaos.

They aren't driven by the need for rapid turnover.

Instead, they are driven by meaning, accuracy, and patient connection.

If this sounds like you, you may be aligned not just with sonography — but with its culture, its pace, its emotional tone, and its purpose.

The Pace and Pressure: Slow Hands, Fast Thinking

The room may be quiet, but the mental pace is fast.

You must:

• interpret images in real time

• adjust angles constantly

• chase elusive anatomy

• differentiate pathology from artifact

• capture images that will direct treatment

• make rapid decisions during trauma or emergent scans

• adapt your scanning plan for each body type

• troubleshoot equipment, patient needs, and clinical questions

You don't have "time to think" later.

You think as you scan.

It is a career where the hands slow down but the mind speeds up.

And that cognitive duality — slow hands, fast brain — becomes addictive to those who love it.

The Technical Work: Machines Are Only as Good as the Person Using Them

The equipment is advanced, but the skill is human.

A sonographer must understand:

• how each transducer works

• how to optimize depth, gain, focus, frequency, and Doppler settings

• how motion affects image clarity

• how to scan around scar tissue or body habitus

• how to capture flow in difficult angles

• how to navigate patients who cannot hold their breath, roll, or remain still

AI is entering imaging, but sonographers remain irreplaceable because:

• no algorithm can replicate human judgment

• no software can sense pain, anxiety, or subtle clues

- no machine can empathize
- no automated pathway can adapt to the infinite variability of real bodies

Sonographers are the interpreters.

The machine is the instrument.

Skill — not hardware — makes the image.

The Lifestyle Realities: What No One Tells You

Every specialty comes with its own lifestyle.

OB/GYN

Emotionally rich, unpredictable, meaningful, sometimes heavy.

Vascular

Methodical, detail-focused, mentally stimulating, consistent.

Echo

Complex, technical, constantly evolving, collaborative with cardiology.

General

High variety, fast turnover, broad anatomy, intellectually diverse.

Breast

Emotionally sensitive, one-on-one, deeply impactful.

Pediatrics

Creative, tender, unpredictable, team-oriented.

Emergency

High-intensity, rapid-response, high-stakes.

Your **alignment** often comes down to matching your inner world with the outer world of your chosen specialty.

The Career Arc: How Sonographers Grow

This profession offers more than a single lane. Career growth can include:

- modality specialization
- teaching
- traveling sonography
- department leadership
- clinical applications specialist
- research imaging
- sonography education
- high-risk maternal-fetal medicine
- pediatric specialization
- advanced certifications in vascular or cardiac imaging
- point-of-care ultrasound (POCUS) leadership
- system quality and standards
- procedural guidance imaging
- mobile/independent practice in some states

It's one of the most flexible imaging careers in healthcare.

The Alignment Truth: Why People Stay or Leave

People stay when:

- the emotional tone matches their temperament
- the schedule fits their life
- the specialty fits their strengths
- the patient population resonates with them
- they feel valued
- the work still feels meaningful

People leave when:

- misalignment grows quietly
- physical strain accumulates
- emotional fatigue is ignored
- the environment becomes unhealthy
- the specialty no longer reflects who they are

This book — and the **SCRUB*fit*™ Healthcare Career Assessment** — are designed to help you see those patterns before they become career-shaping.

Chapter 9
Alignment Snapshot

The SCRUB*fit*™ Alignment Snapshot

Before you can understand *what* a Diagnostic Medical Sonographer does, you need to understand *who thrives in this role*.

Because sonography is not a job you simply perform — it is a job that fits or misfits you at your core.

SCRUBfit™ was built on one central truth:

Healthcare careers rise or fall on alignment —

the match between who you are and where you belong.

Alignment is not personality alone.

It is not skill alone.

It is not passion alone.

Alignment is that almost electric feeling of *"I am built for this."*

And in sonography, alignment matters more than most people realize.

The Precision Pulse Category

Diagnostic Medical Sonographers live in the SCRUBfit™ category known as **The Precision Pulse** — the clinicians who combine:

- pattern recognition
- technical mastery
- emotional steadiness
- quiet leadership
- intuitive problem-solving
- and unwavering focus

They are the **detectives of the body**, noticing subtle changes that others breeze past.

They are the **calmers of chaos**, steadying a frightened patient with nothing but tone and presence.

They are the **artisans of imaging**, shaping clarity out of grainy shadow.

People who thrive in this category almost always carry these traits:

1. Hyper-observant

They notice details others miss — in anatomy, in behavior, in silence.

2. Calm under pressure

Trauma, uncertainty, heartbreak — the room steadies when they enter.

3. Intuitive

They know when something is off even before the image tightens into focus.

4. Patient and meticulous

Ultrasound rewards those who take their time, who adjust, who persist.

5. Empathic but grounded

They care deeply without losing themselves in every scan.

6. Tactful communicators

Sonographers speak truth without speaking diagnosis — a delicate art.

The Alignment Snapshot:

How You Know Sonography Might Be *Your* Work**

If you're reading this because you're curious about the career, here is the internal checklist most future sonographers recognize instantly:

✓ You're drawn to mysteries, puzzles, or hidden patterns.

You like figuring things out.

You like connecting dots.

You like discovering what others overlook.

✓ You prefer impact without the spotlight.

You don't need to be the face of the room to be the force behind it.

✓ You enjoy hands-on, real-time problem-solving.

Not static images.

Not guesswork.

You want to *watch* physiology unfold.

✓ You can be both gentle and firm.

"Can you roll a little?"

"Deep breath again for me."

"Hold still as you can."

Your voice becomes part of the patient's safety.

✓ You are energized by meaningful interactions, not long conversations.

Sonography is intimate and brief — perfect for the empath who doesn't want to be drained by all-day emotional labor.

✓ You have the stamina of an athlete without needing the stadium.

This work is physical — shoulders, wrists, posture, grip.

Alignment includes the body as much as the brain.

✓ You can sit with uncertainty without panicking.

Some scans are joyous.

Some are devastating.

Some are quietly confusing.

A sonographer can manage the emotional weight without letting it fracture them.

Who *Doesn't* Align With Sonography?

Misalignment doesn't mean someone is "bad" at the job — it means the job chips away at them.

People who struggle in this field usually:

- need constant variety rather than deep focus
- prefer long patient interactions
- dislike physical labor
- get overwhelmed by emotional intensity
- want clear-cut, black-and-white answers
- dislike dimly lit, quiet spaces
- need predictable schedules (ultrasound laughs at predictability)
- prefer fast tasks over slow precision

When alignment is wrong, the job feels heavy.

When alignment is right, it feels natural.

The Power of Alignment in Sonography

Aligned sonographers have a very particular energy:

They don't rush.

They don't flinch.

They don't guess.

They don't collapse under pressure.

They don't get lost.

They don't drift.

They move with clarity — physically and emotionally.

And that clarity becomes contagious:

- Patients relax.
- Physicians trust.
- Departments rely on them.
- Chaos softens around them.

Alignment allows sonographers to thrive instead of burn out.

SCRUB*fit*™ Compatibility:

Where Sonographers Overlap With Other Clusters**

Some healthcare careers share DNA with sonography.

When students take the SCRUBfit™ Mini Assessment, sonographers often score close to:

- **Radiology Tech** (The Tech Force)
- **Nuclear Medicine Tech** (Precision + patient interaction)
- **Cardiac Sonographer** (a sibling specialty)
- **Medical Laboratory Scientist** (pattern recognition + precision)
- **Respiratory Therapist** (calm under pressure, acute care clues)

• **Occupational Therapist** (hands-on + intuitive reading of human behavior)

This overlap helps people who love ultrasound build long, adaptable careers — they can specialize, cross-train, or switch zones without abandoning their core alignment.

The Ultrasound Identity

People drawn to sonography always say the same thing:

"I just *knew*. Something about it felt like me."

They don't choose ultrasound.

Ultrasound chooses them.

Because only certain people can step into a dark room, place a hand on someone's abdomen, and translate silence into truth, fear into direction, fear into clarity.

Coming Up Next...

Now that we understand the alignment behind the career, it's time to explore the world sonographers move through every day — the systems, the stakes, the ways ultrasound shapes modern medicine.

Chapter 10

Day in the Life — Emergency Department Sonographer

05:40 — Your alarm goes off and you don't hit snooze because the ER doesn't wait for anyone. You lie still for a beat and run the mental checklist you always run before emergency work: hydration, layers, charged phone, badge, and a breakfast that won't betray you three hours into a shift. Coffee helps, but steadiness matters more. In the emergency department, you don't control the pace, the order, or the emotional temperature of the room—you control your presence inside it.

06:25 — The drive in is quiet enough that it almost feels like you're cheating. The roads are calm. The sky is still figuring itself out. You park, badge in, and walk the familiar hallway into the fluorescent heartbeat of the ED. You can feel it before you see it: rolling carts, overhead pages, the soft urgency in people's voices that never fully turns off.

06:45 — You clock in, grab your machine, and do the first thing that separates a clean shift from a chaotic one: you check your equipment like your day depends on it, because it does. Probe cords, battery, gel, wipes, printer paper, presets, and the one little adapter that always disappears when you need it most. Your department might call you "ultrasound," but in the ED you are also logistics, troubleshooting, and calm under pressure. The charge nurse nods at you on the way by and says, "We've got a list already." Of course you do.

07:05 — First order: right upper quadrant pain, rule out gallbladder. You head to a curtained bay where the patient is trying to act fine, but their hand keeps drifting back to their abdomen like it's magnetized. The lighting is bad, the bed is too high, and the room is crowded with other problems. You introduce yourself, explain what you're doing in plain language, and ask them to breathe the way you need them to breathe—slow in, hold it, let it out—because half of your job is imaging and the other half is coaching people through fear and discomfort without making them feel like a problem.

07:22 — The scan is solid: gallstones, possible inflammation. You capture clean images, annotate, double-check your angles, and send it through. In outpatient imaging, you might have time to perfect. In the ED, you aim for accurate, diagnostic, and fast, because the rest of the chain is waiting on you—labs, meds, surgery consult, disposition. You wipe down your probes, clean the machine, and roll out before the curtain can trap you into a second conversation you don't have time for.

07:48 — The next request hits before you've fully parked: shortness of breath, leg swelling, rule out DVT. You head to another bay and the patient looks tired in a way you recognize —the kind of tired that comes from not being able to catch your breath for days. You work around IV poles and oxygen tubing, finding the best position you can in a room that was never designed for precision. Your hands move steadily while the patient watches your face like it's a weather forecast. You don't promise anything. You just stay calm and do the work.

08:10 — A physician is waiting nearby. Not hovering, exactly, but close. That tells you what kind of scan this is. In the ED, sometimes you are the difference between "we think" and "we know." You finish your compression series, document what you see, and flag the concerning findings. The provider's shoulders tighten just a little, the way they do when a plan becomes urgent. You clean, reset, and move.

08:35 — The trauma pager goes off and the room changes shape. You hear the words before you hear the details: "incoming," "ETA," "high speed," "unstable." You bring your machine toward the trauma bay and suddenly every hallway feels narrower. People who were walking are now moving with purpose. A nurse grabs a warmer blanket. Someone wheels a portable X-ray in like it weighs nothing. You set yourself up where you won't be in the way but you can still work, because trauma is a dance and you need to know your steps without asking for space.

08:52 — The patient arrives and everything is loud. Not just noise—information. Vitals. Mechanism. Meds. Blood. You're asked for a FAST exam. You don't have time to overthink the angles; you have time to be correct. Probe on, gel, window, sweep. You check the places that matter. You look for fluid where it shouldn't be. You hear your own voice calling out what you see, measured and clear, because your tone becomes part of the team's nervous system. If the answer is "negative," you say it like it still matters. If the answer is "positive," you say it like the room can handle it, even if the room is about to erupt into action.

09:20 — Trauma clears out in a wave and leaves behind the aftermath: blood on gloves, used packaging, the smell of adrenaline, and a silence that never lasts. You wipe down your machine carefully because ED equipment touches everything, and everything in the ED is risk until proven otherwise. You restock wipes, restock gel, and glance at the board. The list is longer now.

10:05 — You're called to evaluate early pregnancy bleeding. The patient is young, pale, and doing the brave-voice thing that sounds like confidence until you listen closely. You introduce yourself and speak gently, because this scan isn't just medical—it's existential. You take extra care with your words: you don't narrate findings out loud. You don't speculate. You don't perform reassurance you can't guarantee. You perform steadiness. You get diagnostic images, you document what's needed, and you send it on so the physician can have the hard conversation with the right information in hand.

10:55 — You finally get two minutes to drink water, which you do standing up, because in the ED sitting down is an invitation for the universe to test you. Someone at the desk asks if you can "just squeeze in one more quick one." They always say quick. You always know it might not be.

11:15 — The next scan is renal—rule out hydronephrosis. The patient can't get comfortable, keeps shifting, keeps apologizing for shifting. You tell them they're not doing anything wrong. The scan happens in tiny adjustments: a pillow angle, a breath, a pause, a second attempt. This is what people don't understand about ultrasound: it's not a button you push. It's a skill you apply under imperfect conditions until the image finally gives up what it knows.

12:05 — Lunch exists in theory. You grab a few bites of something you can eat fast, then your phone buzzes again: possible torsion. That one word snaps you back into full focus. You throw your wrapper away, wash your hands, and move.

12:22 — Torsion scans feel like a clock. The patient is in pain, embarrassed about the pain, and scared of what the pain might mean. You keep it clinical without making it cold. You get what you need as quickly as you can without cutting corners. You document, you send, and you walk out knowing you might have just helped save tissue, function, or fertility. You don't celebrate. You just keep moving.

13:10 — Midday in the ED is a strange mix: the morning rush has become a steady stream, and the waiting room is simmering. You get called for IV access support because someone is hard to stick and the team is behind. You bring your machine, switch to vascular settings, and help place a line under ultrasound guidance. It's a small task with a big downstream effect—meds get started, CT gets done, pain gets controlled, the whole machine unblocks a little.

14:05 — A provider flags you down for a bedside echo assessment question. You're not there to replace cardiology. You're there to help the ED answer a time-sensitive problem with the tools available. You position, optimize, capture, and communicate what you can responsibly communicate within your role and protocols. In emergency ultrasound, boundaries matter just as much as speed. You don't wander outside them. You don't guess. You stay precise.

15:00 — The afternoon brings repeat customers: abdominal pain, shortness of breath, swelling, chest discomfort, "I just don't feel right." Your scans stack up. Your legs start to feel it. Your shoulders start to feel it. The ED doesn't care. You adjust your posture, roll your machine, and keep your hands steady anyway.

16:10 — Another trauma call comes in, this one less dramatic but no less serious. You perform another FAST, confirm what you can, and document cleanly. You notice how the newer nurses watch you when you work. Not because you're the main character, but because you look calm and you look sure, and in the ED that kind of presence is contagious. You remember being new and craving that same signal from someone else.

17:05 — The last hour is a push. Not because you're trying to be heroic, but because you're trying to leave the next shift something survivable. You clear your remaining exams, communicate what's pending, wipe down your machine thoroughly, and restock the supplies you always wish someone had restocked for you.

18:00 — You give handoff to the incoming sonographer: the scans you couldn't get to, the patients who were difficult to image, the room that's a mess but has a reason. You don't dramatize it. You just pass truth. Then you clock out.

18:35 — Driving home, the quiet feels too quiet at first. Your brain replays images: the split-second decisions in trauma, the careful silence in early pregnancy bleeding, the way a provider's posture changes when your scan confirms what they suspected. The ED asks you to carry other people's urgency all day and then pretend you can set it down neatly at the door.

20:30 — At home, you eat something simple and try to come back into your own life. Someone asks how your day was and you give the short version because the long version requires context, anatomy, and a tolerance for uncertainty most people don't want at dinner. You shower, you stretch your shoulders, and you feel that specific kind of tired that is half physical and half nervous system.

21:40 — In bed, you think about fit. Emergency department sonography rewards people who can tolerate unpredictability, imperfect conditions, and high emotional temperature without becoming brittle. If you like variety, fast problem-solving, and being useful in the moments when the room is loud and afraid, this work can feel intensely right. If you need quiet control, long setups, and predictable pacing, the ED can slowly grind you down. You fall asleep knowing tomorrow will bring new patients, new puzzles, and the same core truth: in the emergency department, your images don't just show anatomy—they move decisions, and decisions move outcomes.

Chapter 11

Day in the Life — Obstetric (OB) Sonographer

06:10 — Your alarm goes off gently, and unlike emergency imaging shifts, the rhythm of your day will be more structured — but not necessarily lighter. Obstetric imaging carries a different kind of responsibility. Today, many of the people you meet will remember this appointment for the rest of their lives. Some will walk out smiling. Some will leave anxious. A few will receive life-altering news. You remind yourself, as you do every morning, that your role is precision first, compassion always.

07:05 — You arrive at the outpatient women's imaging center, badge in, and greet the front desk staff who are already fielding early arrivals. Expectant parents tend to come early, excited and nervous in equal measure. You check your schedule: first-trimester viability scan, anatomy survey, follow-up growth exam, and two add-on same-day physician requests. A full day, but manageable if the timing holds — which it rarely does.

07:25 — Before the first patient, you prepare the room. You adjust lighting, check probe connections, confirm presets, refill gel warmers, and verify that the printer and image transfer systems are functioning. Ultrasound is as much preparation as performance; a smooth technical setup prevents rushed imaging later when the schedule tightens.

07:45 — Your first patient is early pregnancy confirmation. She looks hopeful but guarded, the way many patients do when they're not sure what they'll hear. You introduce yourself, explain the process clearly, and position the patient comfortably. As the image appears on the screen, you slow your breathing slightly — a habit that keeps your scanning steady. You locate the gestational sac, the embryo, then cardiac activity. Relief washes across the patient's face even before you say a word. You capture the required measurements carefully, document, and let the provider review the results before any official interpretation is shared.

08:30 — The next appointment is a routine anatomy scan, one of the longest and most technically detailed exams of the day. The room fills with quiet anticipation — sometimes partners, sometimes grandparents, sometimes just the patient holding their own nervous excitement. You begin systematically: head structures, spine, heart views, abdominal organs, limbs, placenta, amniotic fluid levels. Every image must meet diagnostic standards, but you also know that many parents are trying to memorize every second. You keep conversation warm but focused; the goal is accuracy first, celebration second.

09:40 — A physician steps in briefly to request additional cardiac views on a patient from earlier in the week. Add-ons happen frequently in obstetric imaging, especially when subtle findings require follow-up. You adjust the schedule quietly, communicating with the front desk to shift the next appointment by a few minutes. Workflow flexibility is an invisible skill in sonography — keeping the day moving without patients feeling rushed or forgotten.

10:15 — A growth follow-up scan requires careful comparison with prior measurements. You review the patient's previous images before beginning, noting fetal position challenges from last visit. Today the fetus cooperates more, allowing clear biometric measurements. You double-check each value before saving. Small measurement differences can influence clinical decisions, and consistency matters as much as precision.

11:30 — Between patients, you sanitize the room, reset linens, and take a quick sip of water. The hallway outside buzzes with quiet conversation — families discussing baby names, appointment times, childcare logistics. The emotional tone of obstetric imaging is different from most specialties: anticipation lives alongside anxiety, and your composure often sets the emotional temperature of the room.

12:05 — A late-morning anatomy scan presents a technical challenge: fetal position limits visualization of key structures. You ask the patient to shift positions, walk briefly, and return. After several attempts, you obtain the necessary images, though the exam runs longer than scheduled. You update the desk so the next patient understands the delay. Communication prevents frustration before it begins.

13:00 — Lunch is short but welcome. In the breakroom, sonographers exchange small tips — which physicians prefer additional Doppler views, which rooms have the most reliable equipment, which time slots tend to run behind. Even brief peer conversations help maintain efficiency across the department.

13:35 — The afternoon includes a high-risk referral requiring detailed imaging. These exams demand heightened concentration: additional measurements, more documentation, and frequent physician consultation. You focus on methodical scanning, ensuring every required view is captured. When the physician reviews the images, you discuss technical aspects briefly — positioning, visualization limits, any repeat images needed — then prepare the room for the next patient.

14:50 — Another routine OB exam follows, lighter in tone. The patient laughs when the fetus stretches dramatically across the screen. Moments like this provide emotional balance during a day that can otherwise carry heavy diagnostic responsibility. You print keepsake images once all diagnostic views are completed, making sure celebration never compromises documentation accuracy.

15:45 — The schedule compresses slightly as earlier delays ripple forward. You maintain steady pacing rather than rushing. Speed rarely saves time if images must be repeated later. Consistency keeps the workflow safer for everyone involved.

16:25 — Your final patient requires a limited follow-up exam ordered urgently by a provider. These short scans often arrive late in the day, and you adjust smoothly, capturing the requested views and communicating completion to the ordering physician. Closing the diagnostic loop before the patient leaves prevents unnecessary return visits.

17:05 — You finish documentation, clean the room thoroughly, and prepare the machine for the next day's team. A well-reset room is a quiet professional courtesy that every sonographer appreciates when their shift begins.

17:35 — Driving home, the emotional mix of the day settles in: the excitement of first-time parents, the technical focus of anatomy imaging, the careful neutrality required when findings are uncertain. Obstetric sonography blends science and human experience in a way few imaging specialties do.

21:10 — As you wind down for the night, you reflect on the rhythm of this specialty. Obstetric imaging rewards sonographers who combine patience, precision, and emotional steadiness. For those who value structured schedules, longitudinal patient care, and meaningful life-event encounters, the role can feel deeply aligned. Each day may look similar on paper, yet every exam carries a different story — and being trusted to document the earliest chapters of those stories is a responsibility few professionals ever experience.

Chapter 12

Day in the Life — Maternal–Fetal Medicine (High-Risk OB) Sonographer

06:05 — Your morning begins earlier than most outpatient imaging schedules because high-risk obstetric clinics run on tightly coordinated physician and diagnostic timelines. Maternal–Fetal Medicine (MFM) imaging is slower, more detailed, and far more consult-driven than routine obstetric scanning. Before leaving home, you mentally prepare for a day that will require both technical precision and emotional steadiness. Many of today's patients will arrive already knowing something may be wrong.

07:00 — You arrive at the MFM clinic, log into the imaging system, and review the day's schedule. Each patient chart includes extensive notes: genetic screening flags, maternal health conditions, prior imaging findings, or referrals from community OB providers. Unlike routine imaging days, the prep time for each patient matters almost as much as the scan itself. Understanding the clinical question guides what you must capture.

07:25 — You power on the ultrasound system, confirm high-resolution presets, check transducers, and ensure all reporting templates are loaded. MFM exams often involve extended measurements, Doppler studies, and detailed fetal anatomy evaluation. Equipment readiness prevents interruptions later when concentration must remain uninterrupted.

07:45 — The first patient is referred for suspected growth restriction. You greet her calmly, explain that today's scan will take longer than standard prenatal imaging, and position her comfortably. As the exam begins, you work systematically: fetal biometry, placental evaluation, amniotic fluid assessment, and umbilical artery Doppler flow. Each measurement is captured carefully and verified before moving forward. Accuracy matters profoundly here — small discrepancies can influence clinical decisions about monitoring or delivery timing.

08:55 — After completing the imaging portion, you briefly confer with the MFM physician, who reviews the images in real time. Collaboration is a defining feature of high-risk obstetric imaging. Sometimes the physician requests additional targeted views; other times the discussion focuses on confirming measurement trends compared with prior studies. You return to the patient to capture the requested images before finalizing the study.

09:40 — The next exam involves detailed fetal cardiac imaging due to abnormal screening results. Cardiac views demand patience and steady probe positioning, especially when fetal positioning is less cooperative. You adjust the patient's position, pause when necessary, and resume imaging once visualization improves. These exams often run longer than scheduled, but rushing never produces usable diagnostic data.

10:50 — Between patients, you document findings, sanitize equipment, and quickly review the next referral note. Many MFM patients arrive anxious, having already received concerning phone calls or referrals. You center your tone carefully when greeting each patient — warm, professional, and steady. Emotional composure is part of the technical skill set in this environment.

11:20 — A consultation case requires serial Doppler measurements to evaluate placental blood flow. The exam is quiet, focused, and methodical. You capture multiple waveform samples to ensure reproducibility and store each dataset according to protocol. When finished, the physician enters the room to speak with the patient, and you step out to prepare for the next exam, giving the provider and patient privacy for discussion.

12:15 — Lunch is brief. In the break area, sonographers discuss subtle imaging challenges from the morning — fetal position difficulties, new protocol updates, equipment calibration notes. In MFM imaging, small technical adjustments shared among colleagues often improve overall departmental quality.

12:50 — The afternoon begins with a twin pregnancy requiring extended imaging time. Multiple fetal assessments, growth comparisons, and placental evaluations require careful sequencing. You maintain steady pacing, ensuring that each fetus is clearly documented and labeled correctly. Accuracy in labeling and measurement prevents downstream reporting errors that can affect clinical interpretation.

14:15 — Another patient arrives for follow-up imaging after a previously detected anomaly. You review prior images before starting, ensuring the same measurement planes are used for comparison. Longitudinal consistency is essential; clinicians rely on trend accuracy more than single isolated values.

15:20 — A physician requests immediate repeat imaging for a patient seen earlier in the day. Add-on scans are common in high-risk clinics, and you adapt the schedule accordingly. Even under time pressure, you maintain the same careful workflow — verify views, confirm measurements, and store images systematically.

16:05 — As the clinic begins winding down, you complete final documentation, verify that all studies transferred successfully to the reporting system, and confirm that any urgent findings were flagged for physician review. Closing administrative loops ensures no patient results are delayed.

16:40 — Before leaving, you clean and reset the room, restock supplies, and prepare the machine for the next day's cases. The next shift depends on the readiness you leave behind, and high-risk imaging clinics rely heavily on that consistency.

17:15 — Driving home, the emotional weight of the specialty sometimes lingers. High-risk obstetric imaging involves both reassuring normal findings and participating in the earliest detection of complex medical conditions. The responsibility is significant, but so is the sense of purpose. For sonographers who value detailed imaging, physician collaboration, and meaningful clinical impact, Maternal-Fetal Medicine can feel deeply aligned — a specialty where precision directly shapes care decisions long before delivery day arrives.

Chapter 13

Day in the Life — General Abdominal Sonographer

06:10 — Your alarm goes off, and you already know the day will involve variety. General abdominal imaging rarely follows a predictable rhythm. Some exams are routine gallbladder studies; others uncover unexpected pathology that shifts the pace of the entire schedule. Over breakfast, you mentally review the common protocol sequences — liver, gallbladder, pancreas, kidneys, spleen — knowing repetition builds speed, but attention to detail keeps patients safe.

07:00 — You arrive in the imaging department, log into the ultrasound workstation, and scan the schedule. The morning includes right upper quadrant pain studies, renal evaluations, and a few complete abdominal exams ordered through the emergency department overnight. You check machine presets, verify probe calibration, and ensure exam templates are loaded correctly before the first patient arrives.

07:25 — The first patient presents with suspected gallstones. After confirming identifiers and reviewing the order, you position the patient and begin imaging the liver before moving to the gallbladder. You adjust breathing instructions to improve visualization, capturing longitudinal and transverse views while documenting wall thickness, shadowing, and surrounding anatomy. Routine studies still require disciplined scanning — small missed findings can change treatment decisions.

08:15 — The next exam involves renal imaging for flank pain. You evaluate both kidneys, capturing cortical thickness, collecting system appearance, and any signs of obstruction. You document ureteral jets when indicated, ensuring the radiologist has the full dataset needed for interpretation. Efficiency grows with experience, but each patient's anatomy requires slight adjustments in technique.

09:05 — A complete abdominal study follows. These exams take longer, requiring systematic evaluation of multiple organs and vascular structures. You move methodically, double-checking measurements and labeling images clearly. In abdominal imaging, labeling accuracy prevents downstream reporting confusion, especially when multiple follow-up studies occur over time.

10:20 — Between patients, you sanitize the room, restock gel and linens, and briefly review the next order. A patient with abnormal liver function tests is scheduled next. You note the clinical indication, which guides additional attention to hepatic texture, bile ducts, and portal vein flow patterns.

10:45 — During the liver-focused exam, you identify an area that requires additional views. You capture supplemental images, documenting the finding carefully without alarming the patient. Maintaining a calm presence while gathering diagnostic-quality images is part of the professional balance of sonography — patients often watch your face closely for clues.

11:40 — Late morning brings a portable request from an inpatient floor. Portable exams introduce different challenges: limited positioning options, crowded rooms, and variable lighting. You transport the machine upstairs, adapt to the environment, and complete the study as efficiently as possible before returning to the department.

12:30 — Lunch is quick. In the break area, sonographers compare notes about schedule flow, challenging body habitus cases, and equipment updates. Informal exchanges often improve department workflow more than formal meetings.

13:00 — The afternoon schedule includes follow-up imaging on a patient with known kidney stones. You compare prior measurements, ensuring that any change in stone size or position is documented consistently. Longitudinal comparison requires replicating measurement planes as closely as possible to maintain reporting accuracy.

14:10 — Another patient arrives with nonspecific abdominal pain. Orders like these require broader scanning coverage. You carefully evaluate multiple organs, recognizing that subtle findings sometimes emerge outside the initial clinical suspicion. Thoroughness prevents repeat imaging later.

15:20 — A stat emergency department order arrives for suspected appendicitis. You prioritize the exam, coordinating quickly with nursing staff to bring the patient to ultrasound. Focused right lower quadrant imaging requires patience and graded compression technique to visualize structures that may be difficult to identify.

16:10 — As the final exams conclude, you verify that all images transferred correctly to the PACS system, complete documentation, and confirm any urgent findings have been flagged for radiologist review. End-of-day verification protects both patients and the department from reporting delays.

16:45 — You clean the room thoroughly, power down unused equipment, and restock supplies for the next shift. Preparation at closing makes tomorrow's start smoother for whoever follows.

17:20 — Driving home, you reflect on how general abdominal sonography blends repetition with unpredictability. Many exams follow familiar protocols, yet each day brings different clinical questions, body types, and diagnostic challenges. For sonographers who appreciate steady workflow combined with ongoing technical problem-solving, this specialty offers a satisfying balance — structured enough to build mastery, varied enough to keep the work engaging.

Chapter 14

Day in the Life — Vascular Sonographer

06:15 — Your alarm sounds before sunrise, and you already know the day will demand sustained concentration. Vascular imaging requires precision, patience, and careful Doppler technique; small measurement differences can influence surgical decisions. Over breakfast, you mentally review the day's likely studies — carotid evaluations, deep vein thrombosis (DVT) exams, and arterial flow assessments.

07:00 — You arrive in the vascular lab, log into the imaging system, and review the schedule. Several carotid duplex studies are booked, along with lower-extremity venous exams ordered overnight from the emergency department. You power up the ultrasound system, confirm Doppler settings, and ensure measurement templates are ready before the first patient arrives.

07:25 — The morning begins with a carotid artery exam. After confirming identifiers and explaining the procedure, you position the patient carefully to optimize neck access. Using grayscale imaging first, you evaluate arterial structure, then activate Doppler to assess blood-flow velocity patterns. Precise angle correction is critical — inaccurate angles can produce misleading velocity readings that affect clinical interpretation.

08:20 — The next patient arrives with symptoms concerning for DVT. You perform a venous compression study, applying gentle pressure along the leg veins while imaging each segment. Lack of vein compressibility can indicate clot presence, making systematic scanning essential. These exams require both technical skill and emotional sensitivity, as patients often arrive worried about serious complications.

09:40 — A peripheral arterial study follows. You evaluate arterial flow through multiple segments of the leg, documenting waveform patterns and velocity changes. Segmental comparisons help physicians determine where narrowing or blockage may exist. You double-check measurements before saving images, knowing treatment plans may depend directly on these numbers.

10:45 — Between patients, you restock supplies and briefly stretch your shoulders. Vascular scanning often involves sustained probe pressure and awkward positioning, making physical endurance part of the profession. Experienced sonographers learn to adjust ergonomics throughout the day to protect long-term musculoskeletal health.

11:10 — Another carotid duplex exam begins, this time on a patient with known vascular disease requiring follow-up comparison. You carefully replicate previous imaging angles and measurement points to ensure accurate longitudinal comparison. Consistency across studies allows physicians to detect subtle disease progression or improvement.

12:05 — Lunch is brief. Conversations in the break room often revolve around complex cases, evolving imaging protocols, and upcoming certification updates. Continuous learning remains essential in vascular imaging as diagnostic standards evolve.

12:35 — The afternoon starts with a dialysis access evaluation. These studies require detailed mapping of fistula or graft flow characteristics, including inflow, outflow, and any stenotic segments. You document flow volumes and waveform changes, ensuring the interpreting physician has comprehensive data for treatment planning.

13:40 — A stat order arrives for suspected arterial occlusion. You reprioritize the schedule and bring the patient in quickly. Focused imaging assesses blood flow to the affected limb, identifying whether perfusion is compromised. Situations like this highlight the direct role vascular imaging plays in urgent clinical decision-making.

15:00 — Later in the afternoon, you complete a venous insufficiency study requiring prolonged standing positions for the patient. These exams take additional time and careful technique, capturing reflux measurements that guide long-term vascular treatment strategies.

16:15 — With the final exam complete, you verify all images and measurements transferred correctly to the reporting system. You review documentation, ensuring urgent findings are appropriately flagged for physician review before leaving.

16:45 — After disinfecting equipment and restocking the room, you power down the system and prepare the lab for the next shift. Small end-of-day steps maintain workflow continuity across the department.

17:20 — On the drive home, you reflect on how vascular sonography blends technical precision with clinical impact. Every angle adjustment, waveform measurement, and carefully labeled image contributes to treatment decisions ranging from medication management to surgical intervention. For sonographers who enjoy analytical imaging, measurable outcomes, and structured diagnostic workflows, vascular imaging offers a career path where meticulous technique directly influences patient care.

Chapter 15

Day in the Life — Echocardiography (Cardiac) Sonographer

06:10 — Your alarm rings early, and before your feet even hit the floor, your mind is already reviewing cardiac anatomy. Echocardiography days require sustained concentration; every chamber measurement, valve image, and Doppler trace may help guide a cardiologist's next clinical decision. You eat a quick breakfast, stretch your shoulders and wrists — small habits that protect you from the repetitive strain common in ultrasound careers — and head to the hospital.

07:00 — You arrive in the echo lab and review the morning schedule. Several transthoracic echocardiograms (TTEs) are booked, along with one stress echo later in the day. You power on the ultrasound system, confirm presets, check ECG lead connectivity, and make sure measurement packages are loaded for efficient workflow.

07:20 — Your first patient is already waiting. After verifying identifiers and explaining the exam, you position the patient in the left lateral decubitus position to optimize acoustic windows. As the probe touches the chest, your scanning sequence begins almost automatically — parasternal long-axis, parasternal short-axis, apical four-chamber, two-chamber, and three-chamber views — each window telling a different part of the heart's story.

08:05 — Doppler imaging follows, capturing blood flow across valves and through cardiac chambers. You carefully align Doppler angles to avoid inaccurate velocity readings. The exam requires both speed and precision; physicians rely on clear measurements of ejection fraction, valve gradients, and chamber size to guide diagnosis and treatment.

09:10 — The next study involves a patient with suspected valvular disease. You spend extra time imaging the mitral and aortic valves, documenting regurgitation patterns and pressure gradients. These exams often demand careful image optimization — adjusting gain, depth, and probe pressure — to capture subtle abnormalities.

10:30 — Between patients, you disinfect the probe, complete measurement packages, and transmit the study to the cardiologist for interpretation. The echo lab runs on steady rhythm: scan, measure, document, reset, repeat.

11:00 — A portable echocardiogram request arrives from the intensive care unit. You transport the machine upstairs, navigating tight hallways and monitoring equipment. Bedside studies require flexibility — limited positioning options, critical-care lines, and urgent clinical questions often mean you must obtain the best possible images under imperfect conditions.

12:10 — Lunch is brief. Echo labs often operate on packed schedules, and urgent add-on studies frequently appear mid-day. You check the afternoon list while finishing your meal, mentally preparing for the stress echocardiogram scheduled next.

12:40 — The stress echo begins. Working alongside the cardiology team, you capture baseline cardiac images, then prepare to image immediately after treadmill exercise. Timing is critical; the window for capturing peak-stress cardiac function is short, and efficiency makes the difference between a diagnostic and nondiagnostic study.

14:00 — The remainder of the afternoon includes follow-up echocardiograms for patients with known cardiac disease. For these cases, consistency matters as much as technique; replicating prior imaging views allows physicians to track disease progression over time.

15:40 — As the final patient leaves, you review completed studies, ensure measurements are finalized, and confirm urgent findings have been flagged appropriately for cardiologist review. Accurate labeling and documentation ensure smooth interpretation later.

16:15 — You disinfect equipment, restock gel and linens, and prepare the room for the next shift. Echo labs depend on careful handoffs, and small end-of-day routines prevent delays tomorrow morning.

17:00 — Driving home, you reflect on the unique role of cardiac sonography. Few diagnostic careers allow clinicians to visualize a beating heart in real time, watching physiology unfold second by second. Each study combines anatomy, physics, clinical reasoning, and patient interaction — a balance that keeps the work intellectually engaging and clinically meaningful. For sonographers who enjoy precision imaging, cardiovascular physiology, and direct clinical impact, echocardiography offers a demanding but deeply rewarding path within diagnostic medicine.

Chapter 16

Day in the Life — Pediatric Sonographer

06:30 — Your morning begins with a slightly different mindset than most imaging days. Pediatric sonography requires not only technical skill but emotional intelligence, patience, and the ability to adapt quickly to children who may be frightened, restless, or unable to follow instructions. Over breakfast, you glance at your schedule: neonatal cranial ultrasound, pediatric abdominal study, and a possible add-on for pyloric stenosis evaluation.

07:20 — You arrive in the pediatric imaging department and prepare your room with extra care. Pediatric probes are smaller, exam presets are adjusted for tiny anatomy, and the room lighting is softened to make the environment less intimidating. A few distraction tools — stickers, small toys, and colorful ceiling projections — are placed within reach.

07:45 — Your first patient is a newborn from the neonatal intensive care unit. A cranial ultrasound is ordered to evaluate possible intracranial bleeding. Working bedside in the NICU, you gently position the probe over the infant's fontanelle, using it as an acoustic window to visualize the developing brain. The exam requires steady hands and quiet efficiency; fragile patients tolerate only limited handling.

08:30 — Back in the imaging suite, a toddler arrives for an abdominal ultrasound. The challenge is not anatomy — it is cooperation. You kneel to the child's eye level, explain the "magic camera," and allow them to hold the gel bottle for a moment. Small gestures often transform anxiety into curiosity, making the exam smoother for everyone involved.

09:40 — The next case is a suspected pyloric stenosis evaluation in a young infant. These studies require precise measurement of the pyloric muscle thickness and channel length. You adjust depth and gain carefully, freezing images at just the right moment to obtain accurate measurements that will determine whether surgery is necessary.

10:50 — Between exams, you disinfect probes, finalize measurements, and communicate any urgent findings to the radiologist. Pediatric imaging often moves quickly, especially when surgical decisions depend on same-day results.

11:30 — A portable ultrasound request comes from the pediatric ward. You transport the machine upstairs to evaluate a patient with possible appendicitis. Bedside pediatric exams require flexibility, working around IV lines, parents at the bedside, and children who may be uncomfortable or frightened.

12:30 — Lunch is short but welcome. Pediatric sonographers often work at a steady pace, balancing technical imaging with the additional emotional energy required to support young patients and their families.

13:10 — The afternoon includes a renal ultrasound for a school-age child. At this age, communication becomes easier; you explain each step and allow the patient to watch the screen. Many children become fascinated when they realize they are seeing images of their own organs in real time.

14:30 — An add-on emergency study arrives from the emergency department. Pediatric emergency imaging requires rapid adaptability — different equipment, unfamiliar staff, and urgent clinical questions. You move efficiently, obtain the required views, and transmit the study immediately for interpretation.

15:50 — With scheduled exams complete, you review images, confirm measurements, and ensure documentation is accurate. Pediatric imaging demands meticulous labeling because anatomy is small and subtle findings can be easily overlooked without careful attention.

16:20 — You clean your room, restock supplies, and prepare equipment for the next shift. Pediatric departments rely heavily on smooth workflow transitions, especially when emergency add-ons are common.

17:00 — On the drive home, you reflect on the unique rewards of pediatric sonography. The technical work is challenging, but the emotional dimension is equally significant. Helping anxious parents find answers, calming frightened children, and capturing diagnostic images in tiny, rapidly changing bodies requires a blend of skill, patience, and empathy that defines this specialty. For sonographers drawn to working with children and families, pediatric imaging offers a career that is both demanding and deeply meaningful.

Chapter 17

Day in the Life — Breast Imaging Sonographer

07:15 — The day begins quietly, but breast imaging carries a different emotional tone than many other ultrasound specialties. Over coffee, you review the schedule: diagnostic breast ultrasounds, a possible biopsy assist, and several follow-up studies. You know many of the patients arriving today are anxious, some returning after abnormal mammogram findings, others waiting for answers that could change everything.

07:50 — You arrive early to calibrate the ultrasound unit, confirm presets for breast imaging, and prepare biopsy trays that may be needed later. Breast imaging requires meticulous setup — correct transducers, measurement protocols, and labeling workflows must be precise because even small documentation errors can create diagnostic confusion.

08:10 — The first patient arrives for a targeted diagnostic ultrasound after a screening mammogram showed an area requiring further evaluation. You introduce yourself calmly, explain the exam step by step, and emphasize that ultrasound is being used to gather more information — not to make assumptions. Patients often watch your facial expressions closely, trying to read clues before results are officially discussed.

08:45 — During the scan, you methodically evaluate the area of concern, documenting lesion size, shape, margins, vascularity, and depth. You capture orthogonal images and measurements exactly as required by breast imaging protocols. Consistency is essential; surgeons and radiologists rely heavily on these measurements when planning next steps.

09:40 — The next study is a short-interval follow-up for a previously identified benign lesion. These exams are often faster technically, but emotionally they remain significant. Many patients arrive expecting reassurance yet still carry lingering anxiety. A calm presence and clear explanations can make a measurable difference in their experience.

10:30 — A radiologist requests your assistance with an ultrasound-guided breast biopsy. You prepare sterile supplies, position the patient carefully, and help maintain visualization of the lesion while the physician performs the procedure. Coordination between sonographer and radiologist is critical; small probe adjustments guide needle placement with millimeter precision.

11:45 — Between cases, you finalize documentation, verify measurements, and ensure images are correctly labeled for the radiologist's review. Breast imaging documentation standards are particularly strict because findings are tracked longitudinally across years of screening and follow-up care.

12:15 — Lunch is brief, and conversations in the break room often reflect the emotional intensity of the specialty. Staff members learn to support one another quietly, recognizing that difficult cases can stay with you longer than the technical aspects of the day.

13:00 — The afternoon begins with a young patient presenting for evaluation of a palpable lump. You explain the process carefully, maintain professionalism, and allow time for questions. Many patients remember not only what the exam showed, but how they felt during the experience — whether they felt rushed, dismissed, or supported.

14:20 — Another diagnostic case requires extensive scanning of multiple breast quadrants and axillary regions. These longer studies demand sustained concentration, careful probe positioning, and consistent image labeling to ensure the radiologist has a complete diagnostic dataset.

15:40 — A final biopsy add-on extends the day slightly. You assist again, maintaining visualization of the lesion while sterile technique is preserved. Even after years in the specialty, these procedures still carry a sense of gravity; every team member understands the importance of precision and calm coordination.

16:30 — With patients finished, you disinfect equipment, complete image reviews, and ensure all measurements and annotations are correct. Breast imaging errors can lead to unnecessary repeat exams or delayed care, so end-of-day quality checks are taken seriously.

17:00 — Driving home, you reflect on the emotional duality of the role. Breast imaging sonographers combine high-level technical skill with constant patient interaction during vulnerable moments. Some days bring reassuring findings; others require guiding patients through the first steps of difficult diagnoses. For sonographers who value meaningful patient interaction and meticulous diagnostic work, this specialty offers a deeply impactful, patient-centered career path.

Chapter 18

Day in the Life — Interventional Procedure Sonographer

06:45 — Your alarm goes off earlier than usual because interventional days require additional preparation. Over breakfast, you mentally review the schedule: two ultrasound-guided biopsies, a paracentesis assist, and a possible add-on drainage procedure. Interventional imaging carries a procedural pace that feels closer to surgery than to routine diagnostic scanning.

07:25 — You arrive in the department and begin equipment checks. Procedure rooms require more preparation than standard ultrasound suites — sterile probe covers, biopsy kits, lidocaine trays, specimen containers, and labeling materials must all be ready before the first patient arrives. You confirm that the ultrasound system is configured for procedural presets and needle-visualization settings.

07:55 — The first patient is being prepared by nursing staff. You review the indication for the biopsy with the radiologist and confirm lesion location, patient positioning, and required supplies. Clear pre-procedure communication helps the room run smoothly once sterile technique begins.

08:20 — After the patient is positioned and prepped, you assist with sterile draping and apply the sterile probe cover. During the biopsy, your role is to maintain constant visualization of the target while the physician advances the needle. Small probe adjustments — sometimes only a few millimeters — help guide accurate placement.

09:15 — Once tissue samples are obtained, you help confirm specimen labeling and imaging documentation. Interventional exams require precise recording of needle paths, lesion measurements, and post-procedure imaging to verify that the targeted area was successfully sampled.

10:05 — The next case involves assisting with an ultrasound-guided paracentesis. You scan the abdomen to identify the optimal fluid pocket while avoiding bowel loops and vascular structures. After marking the site, you continue to monitor fluid drainage using real-time imaging as the physician performs the procedure.

11:10 — Between procedures, you reset the room, dispose of sharps containers, and prepare new sterile fields. Procedure turnover requires attention to infection-control protocols, instrument tracking, and equipment sterilization before the next patient enters.

11:45 — Lunch is shorter on interventional days because schedules often shift with add-on procedures. Conversations with colleagues usually center around workflow coordination — which cases are pending, which rooms are opening next, and whether emergency add-ons are expected.

12:30 — An add-on lymph node biopsy is scheduled for the afternoon. You perform the initial localization scan, documenting measurements and identifying safe needle pathways. Interventional sonography requires strong anatomical awareness; identifying adjacent vessels, nerves, or sensitive structures is essential before any needle enters the field.

13:40 — During the procedure, you maintain needle visualization continuously, adjusting the transducer angle to keep the needle tip visible at all times. Good communication with the radiologist — brief, precise statements such as "needle tip visualized" or "slightly superficial" — helps maintain procedural accuracy.

14:50 — Afterward, you assist with post-procedure imaging to confirm the absence of immediate complications and ensure that the targeted tissue region was adequately sampled. Documentation is finalized quickly so pathology tracking can begin without delay.

15:35 — The final scheduled case involves assisting with a small abscess drainage. Though shorter than earlier procedures, the workflow remains methodical: sterile setup, lesion visualization, drainage monitoring, and post-procedure imaging confirmation.

16:30 — With procedures complete, you disinfect equipment thoroughly, verify that specimen logs match imaging records, and restock sterile kits for the following day. Interventional rooms must remain procedure-ready at all times, and preparation today prevents delays tomorrow.

17:05 — Driving home, you reflect on how interventional sonography blends diagnostic imaging with procedural teamwork. Unlike routine scanning days, procedure days involve constant coordination with physicians, nurses, and technologists. For sonographers who enjoy high-precision imaging, real-time clinical impact, and collaborative procedural environments, this specialty offers a fast-paced and highly technical career path.

Chapter 19

Day in the Life — Mobile Sonographer (Traveling Between Facilities)

05:10 — Your alarm rings earlier than most imaging days because mobile routes start before traffic builds. You check your phone for the day's schedule: three skilled nursing facilities, one outpatient clinic, and a possible afternoon hospital add-on. Mobile sonography is less about staying in one imaging suite and more about bringing imaging wherever patients cannot easily travel.

05:45 — After a quick breakfast, you load the vehicle assigned to your route. The portable ultrasound system is already secured inside its transport mount, but you double-check probe connections, battery levels, gel supply, cleaning wipes, and paperwork. Unlike hospital departments, there is no central supply room waiting if something is missing. Preparation is everything.

06:30 — You arrive at the first skilled nursing facility just as the day shift begins. Staff greet you with a printed patient list and room numbers. Many of these patients cannot be transported easily, which is why mobile imaging services are essential. You begin setting up your portable system in a patient room, adjusting lighting, positioning, and privacy curtains to create the best scanning environment possible.

07:05 — The first exam is a lower-extremity venous study to evaluate for possible deep vein thrombosis. Portable exams require flexibility; beds may not adjust the way hospital stretchers do, and you often work in tighter spaces. You reposition carefully, optimize the image as best as the environment allows, and document your findings before moving on to the next room.

08:10 — The second patient requires an abdominal scan. A nurse helps position the patient, and you adapt again — sometimes scanning seated patients, sometimes scanning with limited mobility or medical equipment surrounding the bed. Mobile sonographers develop strong problem-solving skills because no two exam environments are the same.

09:25 — After completing the facility's patient list, you disinfect the equipment thoroughly, pack up the system, and begin the drive to your next location. Mobile work involves as much travel time as scanning time, and efficient routing helps keep the day on schedule.

10:10 — At the outpatient clinic, the workflow feels closer to a traditional imaging center. You wheel the portable unit into a designated exam room and perform several scheduled exams, including thyroid and soft-tissue imaging. The environment is more controlled than earlier, but you still operate independently, managing both technical performance and patient flow.

12:15 — Lunch often happens in the car between locations. You review your next assignments, upload completed exam data through the secure network connection, and confirm that all patient identifiers and reports have transmitted correctly before moving on.

13:05 — The afternoon includes a hospital call requesting a bedside echocardiogram for a patient who cannot be transported to the cardiology department. You check in at the nursing station, verify the order, and bring the portable system to the patient's room. Hospital bedside imaging requires coordination with nursing staff, monitoring equipment, and occasionally respiratory support devices that shape how you position both patient and probe.

14:30 — With the hospital exam complete, you finalize image uploads and documentation before leaving the facility. Mobile sonographers must maintain strict data-transfer workflows to ensure studies are available quickly for physician interpretation, even when exams are performed miles away from the reading site.

15:45 — The final stop of the day is another long-term care facility with two scheduled exams. Fatigue can build during mobile days, but maintaining consistent image quality remains essential. You repeat the routine: setup, patient identification verification, scanning, documentation, equipment cleaning, and repacking.

17:20 — Once all exams are completed, you return the vehicle to the equipment staging area. Batteries are placed on chargers, probes are disinfected again, and supply levels are restocked for tomorrow's route. A final review of completed exams ensures nothing remains pending for transmission.

18:05 — Driving home, you reflect on how different mobile sonography feels compared to working in a single department. The independence, travel, and variety of patient environments appeal to some sonographers who enjoy autonomy and constant movement. Others prefer the predictability of fixed imaging suites. Either way, mobile imaging plays a vital role in expanding diagnostic access to patients who might otherwise go without timely care.

Chapter 20

Day in the Life — Outpatient Imaging Center Sonographer

06:40 — Your alarm sounds later than hospital shift alarms, one of the quiet advantages of outpatient imaging. The pace will still be steady, but rarely chaotic. You move through your morning routine knowing the day will be scheduled almost entirely by appointment blocks rather than emergency add-ons.

07:45 — You arrive at the imaging center, greet the front desk staff, and review the day's schedule. The list is full: abdominal studies, thyroid exams, pelvic imaging, and several follow-up scans for patients being monitored over time. Outpatient sonography is built around efficiency, consistency, and patient experience.

08:00 — In the ultrasound room, you power on the system, check probe presets, confirm that image archiving is functioning properly, and restock gel, linens, and disinfecting supplies. Unlike inpatient settings, outpatient rooms often run continuously with minimal downtime, so preparation before the first patient arrives is essential.

08:20 — Your first patient arrives early for an abdominal exam. You review their order, confirm preparation instructions were followed, and begin the scan. Outpatient patients often ask more detailed questions about the process because they are fully awake, alert, and engaged in the appointment experience. Calm explanations and clear communication become part of the workflow.

09:15 — The next several patients rotate quickly through the schedule: a thyroid study, a renal exam, and a pelvic ultrasound. The pace is steady but controlled, allowing you to refine technique and maintain consistent imaging protocols. Many outpatient cases are follow-up exams, so comparison imaging and precise measurement documentation are especially important.

11:30 — A physician office calls requesting an urgent same-day appointment for a suspected gallbladder issue. The scheduler fits the patient into an open slot, reminding you that outpatient environments still require flexibility even when most exams are planned.

12:10 — Lunch is brief but predictable. Unlike hospital imaging, outpatient sonographers are more likely to have scheduled breaks that actually occur close to the planned time. You step into the break room, review the afternoon schedule, and return to the scanning suite before the next patient arrives.

13:00 — The afternoon brings obstetric follow-up imaging and vascular screening studies. Many patients are returning for progress checks, and some remember you from prior visits. Outpatient settings often create continuity that hospital-based roles do not always provide, allowing you to see patient progress over weeks or months.

15:20 — The final exams of the day include a musculoskeletal study and another abdominal scan. You complete image labeling, measurements, and preliminary documentation before sending studies for physician interpretation. Accuracy and completeness at this stage prevent delays later in the reporting chain.

16:30 — After the last patient leaves, you disinfect the probes, restock supplies, and review the next day's schedule. Outpatient departments rely heavily on predictable workflow preparation, and leaving the room ready for the next shift supports the entire team's efficiency.

17:05 — You clock out with the feeling of having completed a full day of meaningful patient interaction without the unpredictability of emergency imaging. On the drive home, you reflect on how outpatient sonography offers a rhythm many clinicians value: structured hours, consistent patient flow, and the opportunity to build technical mastery through repetition and refinement.

Chapter 21

Day in the Life — Rural Hospital Sonographer

05:35 — Your alarm sounds early, earlier than many outpatient roles but typical for rural hospital imaging where staffing is lean and coverage often starts before sunrise. You get ready quickly, knowing that today you may scan anything from obstetrics to trauma to vascular studies. Rural sonographers are generalists by necessity.

06:30 — You arrive at the hospital, greet the night shift nurse finishing documentation, and check the imaging worklist. Unlike large systems where departments are highly specialized, the rural list contains a mix: a first-trimester obstetric exam, an abdominal pain evaluation from the emergency department, and a scheduled carotid Doppler study later in the morning.

06:50 — In the ultrasound room, you power on the system, verify probes are clean and functioning, and confirm connectivity with the hospital's imaging archive. Equipment redundancy is limited in smaller facilities, so early equipment checks are essential.

07:15 — The emergency department calls requesting an abdominal scan for a patient with severe right upper quadrant pain. You wheel the portable ultrasound machine to the ED, perform the exam at the bedside, and capture the necessary images while the physician reviews clinical findings nearby. In rural settings, imaging and decision-making often happen side by side in real time.

08:40 — Back in the imaging room, you perform the scheduled obstetric exam. The patient recognizes you from a previous visit; continuity is common in smaller communities. You complete the measurements, capture fetal cardiac activity, and reassure the patient that the images will be reviewed by the radiologist shortly.

10:20 — A physician stops by requesting a quick vascular check for a suspected deep vein thrombosis. Rural sonographers frequently field direct provider requests, sometimes adjusting the schedule to accommodate urgent needs while still maintaining documentation standards.

12:00 — Lunch is flexible rather than guaranteed. Some days allow a full break; other days require eating quickly between exams. Today you manage fifteen quiet minutes in the staff lounge before the pager interrupts with another ED request.

13:10 — A trauma alert arrives from a nearby highway accident. You assist with a focused bedside ultrasound to help evaluate internal bleeding risk while the emergency team stabilizes the patient. The exam is brief but high stakes, and your images contribute directly to immediate clinical decisions.

14:45 — The afternoon returns to scheduled outpatient imaging: renal studies, a thyroid exam, and a follow-up pelvic scan. Switching rapidly between exam types is routine in rural practice, requiring strong cross-specialty competence.

16:20 — Before the end of shift, you review pending imaging, confirm all studies are uploaded correctly, and notify the on-call sonographer about any expected evening cases. Many rural hospitals rely on rotating call coverage, so communication at shift change is critical.

17:05 — You leave the hospital knowing that the day's work ranged across nearly every imaging category. Driving home along quieter roads, you reflect on how rural sonography demands versatility and independence. For clinicians who enjoy variety, autonomy, and strong community connection, this environment can feel deeply aligned with both professional skill and personal purpose.

Chapter 22

Day in the Life — Trauma Center Night-Shift Sonographer

18:30 — Your shift begins as the day team finishes their final reports. Night shift in a trauma center is unpredictable; some nights move steadily, others explode into motion without warning. You review the handoff list, checking for pending studies and any unstable patients who may require overnight imaging.

19:10 — You prepare the ultrasound suites and portable machines, ensuring batteries are fully charged, probes are disinfected, and emergency exam presets are loaded. Trauma centers rely heavily on portable imaging, and readiness often determines how quickly physicians can make critical decisions.

19:45 — The emergency department calls for a focused trauma ultrasound on a patient arriving by ambulance. You bring the portable machine directly to the trauma bay, working around physicians, respiratory therapists, and nurses moving quickly through resuscitation steps. Your images help determine whether internal bleeding is suspected, influencing the next steps of care.

21:00 — A quieter stretch allows you to complete scheduled inpatient exams: a renal Doppler study, a venous thrombosis evaluation, and a bedside abdominal scan for a patient with unexplained pain. Night-shift sonographers frequently cover both emergency and inpatient needs simultaneously.

23:20 — Another trauma alert activates. This time the patient is stable but requires a rapid abdominal and pelvic scan. You move efficiently, capturing images while the surgical team watches the monitor, discussing potential next actions. The atmosphere is calm but intensely focused.

01:05 — Overnight hours often bring cases that could not be completed earlier: ICU follow-ups, transplant checks, and urgent vascular studies. You perform a bedside echocardiographic screening exam requested by a critical care physician evaluating cardiac function changes.

02:30 — A brief lull finally appears. You restock gel bottles, clean probes again, and complete documentation while the department quiets. Night-shift clinicians learn to use calm moments wisely because the next call can arrive at any second.

03:50 — A stat obstetric evaluation is requested for a patient with sudden pain and decreased fetal movement. You move quickly to labor and delivery, perform the exam, and alert the obstetrics team as images are reviewed. Even at night, ultrasound findings can trigger rapid clinical responses.

05:40 — As morning approaches, inpatient orders begin to accumulate. You complete two early-morning vascular studies before the day shift arrives, ensuring the team starts with an updated patient list.

06:55 — You hand off remaining pending cases to the incoming staff, documenting completed studies and any equipment issues. Night shift rarely ends with applause, but the department now begins the day already prepared.

07:20 — Driving home, fatigue mixes with a quiet sense of purpose. Trauma center night work is intense and unpredictable, but for sonographers who thrive under pressure and value being part of critical, time-sensitive decision-making, the role can feel deeply meaningful and professionally energizing.

Chapter 23

Day in the Life — Research / Advanced Imaging Sonographer

06:40 — Your alarm goes off slightly later than many hospital-based roles, but your day requires a different kind of focus. Instead of preparing for a nonstop flow of emergency exams, you'll spend the day working on specialized imaging protocols tied to research studies and advanced diagnostic development. As you get ready, you mentally review today's schedule: two clinical trial patients, one protocol validation scan, and an afternoon session working with engineers testing a new imaging algorithm.

07:45 — You arrive at the medical center's research imaging wing, a quieter environment than the main hospital but filled with its own intensity. After logging in, you review study protocols outlining exactly how each scan must be performed —probe type, measurement sequence, patient positioning, and documentation requirements must match research standards precisely. In research imaging, consistency is as important as image quality.

08:30 — Your first participant arrives, enrolled in a cardiovascular imaging study evaluating early vascular disease markers. You explain the extended imaging process, which takes longer than standard clinical exams, and answer questions about how the images will contribute to long-term research. Many patients feel reassured knowing their participation helps advance future medical care.

09:15 — The scanning session begins. You capture routine vascular measurements first, then proceed through specialized protocol steps, including repeat imaging sequences designed to compare machine-learning detection models with traditional interpretation. Each measurement is recorded with strict labeling requirements so researchers can analyze the data accurately months or even years later.

10:40 — After the exam, you upload imaging files to a secure research database, verifying that all protocol checkpoints were completed. Research work often includes more documentation than clinical practice, but that precision ensures the findings will be scientifically reliable.

11:30 — The second participant requires abdominal imaging as part of a longitudinal liver fibrosis research study. Because repeat scans must be comparable over time, you carefully match probe angles and patient positioning to previous imaging sessions. Small differences in technique can affect the interpretation of long-term disease progression.

12:45 — Lunch often becomes an informal collaboration session with research coordinators, physicians, and imaging scientists. Today, an engineer discusses a new probe design intended to improve image penetration in technically challenging patients. You provide feedback from the scanning perspective—what works in theory sometimes feels very different in real clinical environments.

13:30 — The afternoon is dedicated to equipment validation testing. You run a series of standardized phantom scans—using specialized test objects designed to measure image resolution and consistency—helping the engineering team compare output across software updates. While patients never see this part of the job, these validation steps are critical to ensuring that future clinical scanners deliver accurate results.

15:10 — Before the day ends, you review quality assurance logs, ensuring each research scan meets study standards and that no required measurements were missed. If something looks incomplete, you flag it immediately so coordinators can schedule repeat imaging if necessary.

16:20 — You power down the imaging suite, complete final documentation, and check tomorrow's research schedule. Unlike emergency-driven hospital roles, research imaging days are more predictable, but they require sustained concentration and meticulous attention to protocol detail.

17:00 — Driving home, you reflect on the quieter but meaningful nature of this work. Research sonographers may not see the immediate clinical impact of every scan, yet the images collected today may shape diagnostic standards, treatment pathways, or imaging technologies used worldwide in the years ahead.

Chapter 24

Day in the Life — Lead / Senior Sonographer (Supervisory Role)

06:10 — Your alarm rings earlier than most of your team's, not because you always scan first, but because leadership roles start before the first patient arrives. As you drink your coffee, you glance at the department schedule on your phone: staffing assignments, add-on slots, a student clinical rotation starting today, and one open shift you still need to cover. Leadership in imaging often begins with solving problems before anyone else notices them.

07:00 — You arrive at the imaging department and log into the scheduling system, scanning for overnight updates. A technologist called out sick, and a high-volume vascular clinic is already fully booked. You quickly adjust assignments, moving one experienced sonographer to the vascular room and arranging float coverage for routine exams. Within minutes, the day's stability improves—small decisions that prevent large disruptions later.

07:30 — Morning huddle begins. You review the daily case mix, highlight any complex procedures, and remind the team about a new documentation workflow launching this week. A student sonographer is introduced to the staff, and you assign a mentor for the day. While you still perform clinical scans regularly, a large part of your work now revolves around supporting the performance of others.

08:15 — You step into the scanning room to assist with a technically difficult abdominal study. A newer sonographer asks for help visualizing a challenging structure, and you guide probe positioning and imaging adjustments without taking over the exam completely. Teaching in real time—supporting confidence without replacing the learner—is a skill you've developed over years.

09:30 — Administrative responsibilities pull you back to the office. You review quality assurance reports, checking image quality scores, documentation completeness, and turnaround times. One report flags delayed exam uploads from a specific workstation. You contact IT support and flag the issue before it becomes a department-wide slowdown.

10:45 — A radiologist stops by to discuss protocol adjustments for a new vascular screening program. Together, you review exam timing, measurement standards, and workflow impact. Decisions made at this level affect not only diagnostic accuracy but also how smoothly the department operates for months to come.

12:00 — Lunch is often shorter than planned. Between bites, you respond to staffing emails, approve continuing-education requests, and confirm next month's schedule draft. Leadership means balancing clinical credibility with operational responsibility; both demand attention every day.

13:15 — The afternoon includes performance coaching sessions. You meet briefly with a sonographer preparing for advanced certification, reviewing scan technique improvements and discussing case exposure opportunities that will help them qualify. Helping others grow professionally becomes one of the most rewarding parts of the supervisory role.

14:40 — A sudden surge of add-on exams from the emergency department creates temporary backlog pressure. Rather than assigning extra work blindly, you step into a room and perform several scans yourself, relieving the immediate load while maintaining patient flow. Leadership in imaging often means stepping forward clinically when the system needs reinforcement.

16:00 — Before the end of the shift, you complete department reporting: staffing coverage confirmation, equipment maintenance follow-ups, and tomorrow's preliminary assignments. You double-check that high-acuity studies are properly scheduled and that student rotations have appropriate supervision planned.

17:10 — As you leave the department, the evening team is already scanning steadily. You take a final walk through the work area, checking that rooms are stocked and that the next shift has everything needed to run smoothly. Quiet transitions between teams are often the clearest sign that leadership planning worked.

18:00 — Driving home, you reflect on how your role has changed over time. Early in your career, success meant performing excellent scans. Now, success also means building a department where dozens of exams run smoothly, patients are cared for efficiently, and staff members feel supported enough to grow. The work is different, but the impact is wider —and, in its own way, deeply satisfying.

Chapter 25

The 101™ — Diagnostic Medical Sonographer

Introduction

Every healthcare career has two versions: the brochure version and the lived version. The brochure version tells you what the job is called, how long school takes, and what the salary range looks like. The lived version tells you what your shoulders feel like after scanning for eight hours, how often patients cry during difficult exams, how frequently equipment malfunctions at the worst possible time, and how much emotional intelligence the role quietly demands. The purpose of **The 101™** is to bring those lived-experience realities into the open so that your decision about becoming a Diagnostic Medical Sonographer is grounded in clarity rather than assumption.

Diagnostic medical sonography sits at a unique intersection of technology, anatomy, patient communication, and clinical judgment. Sonographers are often the first professionals to detect abnormalities that later guide life-changing medical decisions. That responsibility can feel energizing for people who enjoy investigative work and visual problem-solving, but it can also feel heavy for individuals who prefer predictable, low-stakes workflows. Understanding how the profession actually functions day to day — including pace, expectations, physical strain, and emotional demands — is essential before committing to training programs or long-term career planning.

The following 101 questions are designed to help you evaluate not only whether you *can* become a sonographer, but whether the daily reality of the profession aligns with your personality, tolerance for uncertainty, communication style, and long-term lifestyle goals. Some questions focus on technical aspects such as certification pathways and exam types. Others address topics that students rarely hear about early enough — ergonomics, scheduling variability, emotional exposure, and workplace expectations. Together, they create a structured reflection tool that allows you to compare your expectations with the actual rhythm of sonography practice across hospitals, outpatient imaging centers, and specialty clinics.

Read these questions slowly. Some may confirm your excitement. Others may introduce concerns you had not previously considered. Both reactions are valuable. Alignment is not about eliminating difficulty; it is about understanding what kinds of difficulty feel meaningful to you and which ones quietly drain your energy over time. By the end of this section, you should not simply know more about diagnostic medical sonography — you should understand more clearly whether the profession fits the way you naturally think, work, and interact with people.

1. What do Diagnostic Medical Sonographers actually *do* all day?

A Diagnostic Medical Sonographer's day is image creation with clinical consequences. You are not "taking pictures." You are acquiring diagnostic evidence—clean, complete, correctly labeled, and captured in the right planes—so an interpreting physician can make a call that holds up under scrutiny. That means you greet the patient, verify identity, confirm the order, and quickly assess what you're walking into: pain level, mobility limits, lines and drains, anxiety, language barriers, and whether this exam is routine or emotionally loaded. Then you position, scan, measure, document, troubleshoot artifacts, and repeat until what you captured answers the clinical question.

You also manage the invisible parts: keeping the room moving, staying on schedule, handling add-ons, communicating with nurses and providers, and knowing when to escalate. Sonographers constantly make micro-judgments about image quality, patient tolerance, and whether something looks "off" enough to warrant extra views. The workflow looks calm from the outside, but inside your head it's pattern recognition, anatomy, physics, and patient care happening at the same time.

2. What's the biggest misconception about sonography?

That it's "easy on the body" and "quiet work." Sonography can be physically punishing and cognitively intense. People imagine dim rooms and gentle scans. Reality can include bedside exams in the ICU, scanning through dressings and pain, awkward angles over stretchers, and long days where you're expected to stay fast without sacrificing accuracy. The misconception matters because it sets students up for surprise fatigue and repetitive strain injuries.

The other misconception is that the machine does the thinking. It doesn't. The machine displays what you earn. Your skill is how you find the right window, optimize the image, and capture the views that prove what's normal—or reveal what isn't. Two sonographers can scan the same patient and produce very different diagnostic value depending on technique, persistence, and clinical instincts.

3. How much patient interaction is there, really?

A lot—often more than people expect. You're one-on-one with patients for 20–60 minutes at a time, and you're usually the person physically closest to them during a vulnerable moment. You explain what you're doing, reposition them, manage discomfort, and set expectations. You also read the room: someone who wants every detail versus someone who is terrified and needs calm brevity.

And sometimes you are present for emotionally heavy exams—pregnancy complications, suspected cancer, vascular compromise, trauma. You often can't say what you're seeing, but patients can read your face, your pauses, your re-scans. That means emotional self-control is part of the job. If you dislike conversation, reassurance, or navigating fear in real time, the constant human contact can drain you even if you love the technical side.

4. How physically demanding is sonography, day to day?

More demanding than most healthcare students realize. The strain comes from repetition and posture: sustained shoulder elevation, wrist and thumb overuse, leaning across beds, twisting to reach a window, and holding pressure on the transducer while maintaining image stability. Add portable exams—pushing heavy machines, working around equipment, scanning in tight spaces—and you can see why burnout in sonography often starts as pain.

Ergonomics isn't "extra"; it's career survival. Technique, table height, patient repositioning, micro-breaks, and knowing when to ask for help are not small habits—they decide whether you can do this for ten years without chronic injury. A program can teach you anatomy and physics, but a career teaches you that your body is part of your equipment, and it has limits.

5. Do sonographers interpret results, or only capture images?

In most settings, sonographers are not the final interpreting provider, but the job absolutely requires interpretation-level thinking while you scan. You must recognize what's normal and what's suspicious so you can capture the right additional views, measurements, and Doppler information before the patient leaves. If you miss a key view, the radiologist or cardiologist can't "fix it later." They can only read what you brought them.

In practice, strong sonographers develop a disciplined internal process: confirm anatomy, verify laterality, document measurements, and pursue abnormalities until you have enough evidence to support a confident interpretation by the physician. You're not writing the final impression, but your skill determines whether the exam is diagnostic or wasted time.

6. How fast-paced is it—hospital vs outpatient?

Hospital sonography can be unpredictable and interruption-heavy. You may have a schedule, but add-ons from the ED and inpatient floors can rewrite your day. You might jump from a routine abdominal exam to a stat DVT study, then get called for a bedside scan in the ICU. Speed matters, but so does thoroughness under pressure.

Outpatient imaging centers tend to be more predictable, but productivity expectations can be intense—tight appointment slots, minimal downtime, and pressure to keep the conveyor belt moving. The pace is different, not necessarily easier. If you like variety and can tolerate chaos, hospital work may fit. If you prefer predictable flow and you're okay with higher volume and repetition, outpatient may fit better. Neither environment tolerates sloppy images.

7. What are the common specialties within sonography?

Specialties shape your whole lived reality: what you scan, how long exams take, what emotional situations you see, and what your physical strain looks like. Common lanes include general/abdominal, OB/GYN, maternal-fetal medicine, vascular, echocardiography, pediatric, breast, and procedure guidance. Some sonographers stay broad; others become deeply specialized and build a reputation in one service line.

The important part isn't the list—it's the tradeoff profile. OB can be emotionally intense and high-stakes in a different way than vascular. Vascular can involve heavy call burden and urgent ED add-ons. Echo can be fast-paced with complex interpretation demands. Pediatrics requires patience and creativity with movement and fear. Specialty choice is one of the biggest alignment levers in this career.

8. What education paths actually get you hired?

Most sonographers come through accredited programs (certificate, associate, or bachelor's), with clinical training as the real proving ground. Employers want proof you've scanned real patients under supervision and can produce diagnostic-quality studies safely. The degree matters, but clinical competence matters more.

If you're choosing a program, pay attention to clinical site quality, modality exposure, pass rates, and how well graduates get placed. The shortcut danger is ending up in a program that checks boxes but doesn't produce confidence or competence. Sonography is not forgiving when you're alone with a patient and a machine and the window is hard to find.

9. Is certification required—and how much does it matter?

Even when it's not required by state law, certification is often the difference between "maybe" and "hire." Credentials signal standardized competency and reduce perceived risk for employers. In competitive markets, being uncredentialed can keep you stuck in limited roles or lower-paying environments.

But certification isn't just a hiring checkbox. The process forces you to learn the language of the profession—physics, anatomy, protocols, pathology patterns—and that foundation protects you in practice. It also affects mobility: if you want to switch states, change employers, or move into a specialty later, credentials make those pivots smoother.

10. What kind of person tends to thrive in sonography?

People who thrive tend to share a few traits: patience, visual-spatial thinking, comfort with technology, and a calm communication style. You need the discipline to follow protocols while also having the curiosity to chase an abnormality until you're confident the exam answers the question. You also need emotional steadiness—being present with patients in fear without absorbing everything they're carrying.

If you love precision, pattern recognition, and the satisfaction of building a clean diagnostic story from raw anatomy, sonography can feel deeply right. If you hate repetition, dislike patient interaction, or struggle with sustained physical posture and focus, the job can quietly grind you down even if you think the images are cool.

11. How much autonomy do sonographers have during exams?

Sonographers often work with more real-time autonomy than students initially expect. Once the order is verified and the clinical indication is clear, the sonographer typically determines the sequence of views, adjusts protocols when anatomy or patient tolerance requires flexibility, and decides when additional images are necessary to fully answer the clinical question. While physicians ultimately interpret the exam, the sonographer's judgment shapes the quality and completeness of what the physician sees.

This autonomy is paired with responsibility. If a critical structure is missed, mislabeled, or inadequately documented, the diagnostic chain weakens immediately. Strong sonographers develop a disciplined internal checklist—confirming laterality, verifying measurements, ensuring proper labeling, and reviewing images before sending the study—so that independence does not become inconsistency.

12. What is the most stressful part of the job for new sonographers?

For many new sonographers, the greatest stress is the moment when they realize they are the only person in the room responsible for capturing the images that will drive medical decisions. Early in the career, the pressure to work quickly while still learning scanning techniques can feel intense. Add to that the emotional situations—patients in pain, worried families, or exams where abnormal findings are suspected—and the learning curve becomes both technical and psychological.

Confidence grows with repetition, but the early phase requires resilience. The most successful new graduates are those who ask questions, review their exams critically, and accept that speed naturally improves after accuracy becomes reliable.

13. How important is anatomy knowledge in daily practice?

Anatomy knowledge is foundational. Sonographers must visualize organs in multiple planes, recognize normal variations, and quickly identify when structures appear distorted, displaced, or abnormal. Unlike static textbook diagrams, real patients present with surgical histories, body habitus differences, or disease processes that change expected appearances.

Strong anatomical understanding allows sonographers to adjust probe positioning creatively when the "textbook window" does not work. Without that knowledge, exams become slower, less confident, and potentially incomplete.

14. How often do sonographers interact with physicians?

Interaction levels vary by setting, but collaboration is frequent. Sonographers may communicate with radiologists, cardiologists, vascular surgeons, emergency physicians, or obstetricians to clarify orders, discuss technical challenges, or confirm whether additional images are needed. In some departments, interpreting physicians review studies in real time and provide immediate feedback; in others, communication occurs through electronic notes or follow-up conversations.

Professional communication skills matter. Clear, concise exchanges help physicians interpret studies efficiently and build trust in the sonographer's technical judgment.

15. What role does ultrasound physics play in everyday work?

Ultrasound physics is not just an academic requirement—it is a daily operational tool. Understanding gain, depth, frequency, and Doppler settings allows sonographers to optimize images quickly and reduce artifacts. When images appear unclear, physics knowledge guides troubleshooting: adjusting probe angle, switching frequencies, or modifying machine settings to improve visualization.

Sonographers who understand the physics behind the technology often work faster and produce more consistent diagnostic-quality exams because they know *why* adjustments work, not just *which buttons to press.*

16. How repetitive is the work?

Repetition exists, particularly in high-volume departments where certain exams are performed frequently. However, repetition does not necessarily mean monotony. Each patient presents unique anatomical challenges, clinical histories, and positioning limitations, requiring small adaptations in technique. Over time, repetition builds scanning efficiency and pattern-recognition speed, allowing experienced sonographers to complete exams smoothly while maintaining quality.

For individuals who enjoy refining technical skill through repetition, the workflow can feel satisfying. For those who require constant novelty, repetition may feel draining unless balanced by specialty diversity.

17. How much documentation is required?

Documentation is a core component of the role. Sonographers record measurements, annotate images, confirm exam completeness, and ensure that all required protocol elements are captured before the study is finalized. Proper labeling—laterality, anatomy, and measurement placement—is essential for accurate physician interpretation and long-term medical record clarity.

Incomplete documentation can lead to repeat exams, delayed diagnoses, or billing complications, making attention to detail a professional expectation rather than an administrative afterthought.

18. Do sonographers work independently or always within a team?

Sonographers operate in both modes. Much of the scanning process is performed independently in the exam room, requiring self-direction and problem-solving. At the same time, the broader workflow is team-based, involving schedulers, nurses, physicians, technologists, and administrative staff who coordinate patient flow and care decisions.

Success in the role depends on the ability to function confidently alone while communicating effectively within a clinical team structure.

19. How much continuing education is expected?

Continuing education is an ongoing professional responsibility. Credential maintenance typically requires periodic continuing education credits, encouraging sonographers to remain current with evolving imaging techniques, updated protocols, and technological advancements.

Many professionals also pursue additional specialty credentials over time, expanding both competence and career mobility.

20. Can sonographers advance professionally without leaving clinical practice?

Yes. Advancement does not always require moving into management. Experienced sonographers often become lead technologists, specialty experts, clinical instructors, quality assurance coordinators, or advanced modality specialists. Others expand into education, equipment training, research imaging, or multi-modality roles that combine ultrasound with other imaging technologies.

Career growth in sonography often follows expertise development rather than purely hierarchical promotion, meaning clinical mastery itself can open doors to leadership and teaching opportunities.

21. How important is speed compared to accuracy in sonography?

Accuracy always comes first. While departments maintain productivity expectations, diagnostic imaging depends on capturing the correct anatomy, measurements, and views. An exam performed quickly but incompletely often requires repeat imaging, creating more delays than it prevents.

As sonographers gain experience, speed improves naturally because probe positioning, protocol flow, and machine adjustments become instinctive. Early in the career, the focus should remain on accuracy, completeness, and image quality; efficiency follows with repetition.

22. What types of patients do sonographers work with most often?

Sonographers work with a wide range of patients, including emergency department patients, hospitalized individuals, pregnant patients, outpatients scheduled for routine evaluations, and critically ill patients who cannot easily be transported. Age ranges span from newborns to elderly adults, meaning patient interaction styles must adapt constantly.

Flexibility in communication—explaining procedures clearly to anxious patients, comforting those in pain, and working efficiently with critically ill individuals—is a daily requirement.

23. How often do sonographers encounter unexpected findings?

Unexpected findings occur regularly. Many exams are ordered to "rule out" a condition, and occasionally imaging reveals abnormalities that were not anticipated. When this happens, the sonographer's role is to remain professional, complete the required imaging protocol, and notify the interpreting physician if immediate review is needed.

Emotional composure is essential. Patients may ask questions when they sense concern, and the sonographer must respond with reassurance while avoiding diagnostic interpretation.

24. What is the most important technical skill to develop early?

Probe control is one of the most critical early skills. Subtle changes in pressure, angle, and positioning dramatically affect image quality. Learning how to maintain steady hand positioning while adjusting depth, gain, and focal zones simultaneously allows sonographers to obtain clearer diagnostic images.

Strong probe control reduces exam time, improves consistency, and minimizes patient discomfort, making it a foundational professional skill.

25. How predictable are daily schedules?

Schedules vary by setting. Outpatient imaging centers typically operate on structured appointment blocks, creating more predictable workflows. Hospital departments, particularly those supporting emergency and inpatient services, experience frequent add-on exams and schedule changes throughout the day.

Individuals who prefer structured routines may gravitate toward outpatient settings, while those comfortable with shifting priorities often adapt well to hospital environments.

26. How important is communication with patients during exams?

Communication is central to exam success. Patients who understand what is happening are more likely to remain still, follow breathing instructions, and tolerate positioning that may otherwise feel uncomfortable. Calm, clear explanations also reduce anxiety, which can improve image quality and shorten exam duration.

Strong communication skills often distinguish technically competent sonographers from exceptional ones.

27. How often do sonographers move or transport equipment?

In many hospital settings, sonographers push portable ultrasound machines between departments, patient rooms, and emergency areas. Transporting equipment safely and efficiently is a routine part of the job, particularly during bedside exams.

Over time, repeated equipment movement contributes to the physical demands of the profession, reinforcing the importance of ergonomic technique and body mechanics.

28. Do sonographers specialize early in their careers?

Some begin in general imaging roles and later pursue specialties such as vascular, cardiac, or obstetric sonography. Others enter specialty-focused positions earlier, particularly in larger health systems with dedicated imaging departments.

Specialization often increases earning potential, professional recognition, and scheduling consistency, but it may also narrow the variety of daily cases.

29. How does technology continue to change the profession?

Ultrasound technology evolves continuously, introducing improved image resolution, advanced Doppler capabilities, automated measurement tools, and integration with electronic medical record systems. Sonographers must adapt to new equipment interfaces and workflow enhancements throughout their careers.

Professionals who stay comfortable learning new technology often maintain stronger long-term career flexibility.

30. What makes some sonographers stand out professionally?

Attention to detail, strong patient interaction skills, consistent image quality, and the ability to anticipate physician needs all contribute to professional reputation. Sonographers who communicate clearly, assist colleagues during busy periods, and maintain calm efficiency during complex exams are often viewed as highly reliable team members.

Over time, these qualities influence promotion opportunities, specialty training invitations, and leadership roles within imaging departments.

31. How long does it usually take to feel comfortable working independently?

Most new sonographers begin to feel more comfortable within six to twelve months of full-time practice, though confidence continues to build for several years. Early months involve learning department-specific protocols, machine presets, physician preferences, and workflow pacing.

Independence develops when image acquisition becomes instinctive and the sonographer can adapt exam strategies when patients present with challenging anatomy, mobility limitations, or urgent clinical conditions.

32. How much documentation is required after each exam?

Documentation requirements vary by facility but typically include entering exam measurements, labeling images accurately, verifying patient identifiers, and completing technical worksheets or electronic reports. While documentation may take only a few minutes per exam, accuracy is critical because physicians rely on these records during interpretation and clinical decision-making.

33. Are mistakes common early in the career?

Learning curves are expected. Early mistakes usually involve workflow navigation, machine settings, or incomplete image sets rather than clinical judgment errors. Strong departments provide mentoring and image review processes that help new sonographers improve quickly.

The most effective professionals respond to feedback constructively and treat early challenges as skill-development opportunities rather than setbacks.

34. What types of environments feel most stressful for sonographers?

High-volume emergency departments, trauma centers, and understaffed hospital units often create the most stressful conditions because exam requests arrive unpredictably and time pressures are high. Outpatient centers may feel less chaotic but can still generate stress through tight scheduling expectations and productivity targets.

Stress tolerance varies by personality; some professionals thrive in rapid-response environments, while others prefer structured workflows.

35. How important is teamwork in sonography departments?

Teamwork is essential. Sonographers coordinate constantly with nurses, physicians, transport staff, schedulers, and fellow imaging professionals. Cooperation during busy periods—helping colleagues finish urgent exams or assisting with equipment movement—keeps departments functioning efficiently.

Facilities known for strong teamwork cultures often experience higher retention and lower burnout among imaging staff.

36. Do sonographers ever specialize later in their careers?

Yes. Many sonographers begin in general imaging and later pursue specialty certifications such as vascular, cardiac (echocardiography), obstetrics and gynecology, pediatric imaging, or breast imaging. Specialization can expand clinical responsibility, increase professional marketability, and sometimes lead to higher compensation depending on regional demand.

37. How does shift scheduling typically work?

Scheduling varies widely by setting. Hospitals often require rotating shifts, weekends, holiday coverage, and on-call assignments for emergency imaging needs. Outpatient imaging centers usually operate on more predictable weekday schedules but may still include occasional extended hours to accommodate patient demand.

38. How often do sonographers interact directly with physicians?

Interaction occurs frequently, especially in hospital environments. Sonographers may communicate directly with radiologists, cardiologists, obstetricians, or emergency physicians to clarify exam priorities, confirm additional imaging views, or alert providers to urgent findings that require immediate review.

39. What skills improve scanning efficiency without sacrificing quality?

Efficiency improves through strong anatomical knowledge, consistent probe positioning techniques, familiarity with machine presets, and the ability to anticipate which additional views physicians commonly request. Experience allows sonographers to adjust scanning approaches quickly when patient anatomy or clinical conditions create technical challenges.

40. What is the biggest surprise many new sonographers experience after starting the job?

Many are surprised by how physically demanding the work becomes over time. Sustained shoulder positioning, repetitive arm movements, and frequent equipment movement can create fatigue and musculoskeletal strain if ergonomic techniques are not consistently practiced. Long-term career sustainability depends heavily on early attention to posture, scanning mechanics, and body-preservation habits.

41. How quickly do productivity expectations increase after hiring?

Most departments provide a brief orientation period where new sonographers learn protocols, documentation systems, and equipment layout. However, productivity expectations usually increase within the first three to six months. Once supervisors are confident in scanning accuracy and workflow familiarity, exam volume expectations begin to match those of experienced staff. This transition can feel abrupt for some new hires, especially in high-volume hospitals where schedules are tightly structured. Learning to maintain both speed and diagnostic quality simultaneously becomes one of the earliest professional challenges. Sonographers who develop efficient scanning routines, organized documentation habits, and clear communication with scheduling teams often adjust more comfortably as expectations rise.

42. How much autonomy do sonographers have during examinations?

Diagnostic medical sonographers function with significant procedural autonomy. While interpreting physicians ultimately review the images, sonographers independently determine scanning approach, patient positioning adjustments, image optimization settings, and whether additional views are necessary to clarify findings. During many exams, physicians are not present, meaning the sonographer's judgment directly affects diagnostic completeness. This autonomy requires strong anatomical knowledge, pattern recognition, and clinical awareness to identify abnormalities that require expanded imaging. Over time, experienced sonographers develop the confidence to modify scanning protocols when necessary, ensuring that studies provide physicians with the most complete diagnostic information possible while still maintaining efficiency.

43. What role does continuing education play in long-term success?

Continuing education plays a central role in maintaining certification, improving technical expertise, and adapting to advances in imaging technology. Ultrasound systems evolve rapidly, introducing new software capabilities, imaging techniques, and specialty applications that require ongoing training. Many credentialing organizations require continuing education credits for certification renewal, reinforcing the expectation that professionals remain current throughout their careers. Sonographers who regularly attend workshops, professional conferences, and specialty training programs often gain access to advanced scanning techniques and expanded career opportunities. Over time, continuous learning supports both professional mobility and clinical confidence, helping practitioners remain competitive in a field that increasingly values specialization.

44. How does working in outpatient imaging differ from hospital-based sonography?

Outpatient imaging centers typically offer more predictable scheduling, fewer emergency interruptions, and a narrower range of exam types. Patients generally arrive for scheduled studies, allowing departments to maintain structured workflows. Hospital-based sonography, in contrast, involves greater exam variety, frequent add-on requests, and higher-acuity patient populations, including emergency and inpatient cases. These environments often require rapid room turnover and adaptability as priorities shift throughout the day. While outpatient roles may provide more stable routines, hospital settings often accelerate early-career learning by exposing sonographers to complex clinical scenarios. Choosing between these environments often depends on individual preferences regarding pace, variety, and stress tolerance.

45. Do sonographers need strong computer skills?

Yes. Modern ultrasound systems operate through sophisticated digital interfaces that require familiarity with imaging presets, measurement software, reporting platforms, and electronic medical record integration. Sonographers must routinely adjust imaging parameters, annotate studies, archive images correctly, and ensure accurate patient documentation. Basic troubleshooting skills are also valuable when equipment malfunctions or connectivity issues arise. Professionals who are comfortable navigating technology often complete exams more efficiently and experience fewer workflow delays. As healthcare continues to digitize clinical documentation and imaging storage systems, technical proficiency with software platforms is becoming just as important as hands-on scanning skill.

46. How important is patient communication during exams?

Patient communication is a critical component of successful sonography practice. Many patients arrive anxious, uncomfortable, or uncertain about what the procedure involves, and the sonographer often becomes the primary person guiding them through the experience. Clear explanations of positioning, expected sensations, and exam duration help reduce anxiety and improve cooperation, which directly influences image quality. Compassionate communication also becomes especially important during emotionally sensitive exams, such as pregnancy complications or cancer-related evaluations. Sonographers who balance technical efficiency with calm, respectful patient interaction often contribute significantly to both patient satisfaction and smoother clinical workflow.

47. Can sonographers move into leadership positions?

With experience, many sonographers advance into roles such as lead technologist, department supervisor, clinical educator, or imaging program instructor. Leadership pathways often require demonstrated clinical expertise, reliability, communication skills, and an interest in mentoring newer staff members. Some professionals pursue additional education in healthcare administration or management to prepare for supervisory responsibilities. Leadership roles frequently involve scheduling oversight, quality improvement initiatives, equipment purchasing decisions, and workflow planning. Sonographers who develop organizational and interpersonal leadership skills early in their careers often position themselves for long-term advancement beyond purely technical roles.

48. What types of facilities employ diagnostic medical sonographers?

Diagnostic medical sonographers work across a wide range of healthcare environments, including hospitals, outpatient imaging centers, physician specialty clinics, mobile imaging companies, research institutions, and academic medical centers. Each setting presents different workflow demands and patient populations. Hospitals often offer the greatest variety of exam types and acuity levels, while outpatient centers emphasize efficiency and predictable scheduling. Mobile imaging services require travel between facilities and adaptability to changing equipment setups. Understanding these environment differences helps professionals choose workplaces that align with their pace preferences and long-term career goals.

49. How often do sonographers handle urgent or unexpected cases?

Hospital-based sonographers frequently encounter urgent imaging requests from emergency departments, inpatient units, and surgical teams. These cases may involve trauma evaluations, suspected internal bleeding, vascular emergencies, or critical obstetric situations requiring immediate imaging. Because these requests can arise without warning, sonographers must quickly adjust schedules, prepare rooms rapidly, and perform accurate imaging under time pressure. This aspect of the profession contributes to both the intellectual challenge and emotional intensity of hospital-based sonography roles. Professionals who remain calm under pressure and maintain strong scanning fundamentals often perform most effectively in these high-demand situations.

50. What makes some sonographers advance faster than others?

Career advancement often depends on more than years of experience alone. Sonographers who demonstrate technical consistency, willingness to learn new specialties, strong teamwork behavior, and reliability during high-demand situations tend to progress more quickly. Departments value individuals who can cross-train across exam types, assist during staffing shortages, and contribute positively to team culture. Professionals who actively pursue additional certifications, volunteer for quality improvement projects, or mentor new staff frequently become early candidates for leadership or specialty assignments. Advancement is typically driven by adaptability, initiative, and sustained professional performance rather than tenure alone.

51. How long does it usually take to feel confident in scanning independently?

Most new sonographers begin to feel comfortable with routine examinations within the first six to twelve months of practice, though true confidence often develops over several years. Early in the career, many scans require deliberate concentration as practitioners mentally review anatomy, imaging angles, and measurement techniques. With repetition, muscle memory develops, allowing sonographers to focus more on recognizing subtle abnormalities rather than basic scanning mechanics. Confidence also grows as professionals encounter a wider variety of patient presentations and clinical scenarios. Exposure to different body types, pathology patterns, and workflow challenges gradually builds the judgment needed to perform exams efficiently while maintaining diagnostic accuracy.

52. How does shift scheduling typically work in sonography departments?

Scheduling varies significantly depending on the facility. Hospitals frequently operate with rotating shifts that include evenings, weekends, holidays, and on-call responsibilities, ensuring imaging coverage for emergency and inpatient needs. Outpatient centers usually maintain daytime weekday schedules, offering more predictable hours but often with tightly structured appointment volumes. Some departments allow self-scheduling or shift bidding based on seniority, while others maintain fixed rotations. Understanding the scheduling structure during the hiring process is important because shift expectations directly influence work–life balance, sleep patterns, and long-term job satisfaction.

53. What types of equipment maintenance responsibilities do sonographers have?

Although biomedical engineering departments handle major repairs, sonographers are responsible for routine equipment care, including cleaning transducers, inspecting cables for wear, ensuring proper machine calibration checks, and reporting performance concerns. Proper maintenance practices directly affect image quality and patient safety. Sonographers must also understand infection-control protocols when disinfecting probes used in invasive or high-risk procedures. Maintaining equipment readiness reduces workflow interruptions and helps extend the lifespan of costly imaging systems, making attention to equipment care an important professional responsibility.

54. How does patient diversity affect scanning techniques?

Patients vary widely in body habitus, mobility limitations, age, medical condition, and tolerance for positioning, requiring sonographers to adapt scanning techniques constantly. Adjustments in patient positioning, probe pressure, imaging angles, and machine settings are often necessary to obtain diagnostic images. Pediatric patients, critically ill individuals, or patients experiencing pain may require modified approaches and additional patience. Developing flexibility in scanning technique allows sonographers to consistently produce diagnostic-quality studies even under challenging conditions, reinforcing the importance of technical adaptability throughout the career.

55. How important is teamwork in the sonography profession?

Sonography is deeply collaborative. Sonographers coordinate with physicians, nurses, transport staff, schedulers, and other imaging professionals to ensure exams occur at the right time and in the correct clinical context. Clear communication helps prevent delays, reduces patient confusion, and supports accurate diagnostic interpretation. In hospital settings, teamwork becomes especially critical when urgent exams must be completed quickly to guide treatment decisions. Professionals who communicate effectively, assist colleagues when workloads surge, and maintain cooperative relationships across departments often experience smoother workflows and stronger professional reputations.

56. What are the most common causes of early career burnout in sonography?

Early-career burnout often develops from a combination of physical strain, high productivity expectations, emotional exposure to difficult diagnoses, and irregular shift schedules. New sonographers sometimes underestimate the cumulative effect of repetitive scanning movements and long hours spent performing technically demanding exams. Additionally, adjusting to clinical responsibility while still building confidence can create mental stress. Departments that provide supportive mentoring, ergonomic training, and realistic onboarding expectations help reduce burnout risk. Individuals who prioritize physical conditioning, posture awareness, and healthy recovery habits also tend to sustain longer, healthier careers.

57. Can sonographers specialize later in their careers?

Yes. Many sonographers begin in general imaging and later pursue advanced certifications in specialties such as vascular imaging, echocardiography, breast imaging, or maternal-fetal medicine. Specialty certification often requires additional clinical experience, structured exam preparation, and credentialing examinations. Specialization can increase professional marketability, expand clinical responsibilities, and in some cases improve earning potential. Choosing a specialty often depends on personal interests, department needs, and long-term career goals, making early exposure to multiple exam types valuable when exploring future directions.

58. How does documentation impact workflow efficiency?

Accurate and timely documentation is essential because exam findings, measurements, and technical notes guide physician interpretation and influence patient care decisions. Inefficient documentation habits can slow department throughput and increase reporting delays. Many sonographers develop structured routines for labeling images, completing worksheets, and entering measurements in real time during the exam, reducing the need for later corrections. Mastering documentation systems early in the career often improves overall workflow speed and reduces administrative stress during busy shifts.

59. What role does critical thinking play during examinations?

Critical thinking allows sonographers to adjust imaging approaches when initial views do not fully answer the clinical question. If unexpected findings appear, the sonographer must determine which additional views or measurements are necessary to clarify the situation. This ability to recognize when standard protocols are insufficient and expand the examination appropriately is a key professional skill. Over time, repeated exposure to diverse pathology patterns strengthens diagnostic intuition and improves decision-making speed during complex exams.

60. How does the learning curve change after the first few years in practice?

During the first few years, learning focuses heavily on technical scanning proficiency and workflow familiarity. As experience grows, the learning curve shifts toward recognizing subtle pathology, refining efficiency, and expanding into specialty exams. Experienced sonographers often report that while the physical mechanics of scanning become easier, the intellectual challenge of interpreting complex imaging patterns continues to evolve throughout the career. Ongoing exposure to new technologies, advanced imaging techniques, and emerging clinical protocols ensures that professional growth remains continuous rather than plateauing after initial training.

61. How does experience influence scanning speed without sacrificing accuracy?

As sonographers gain experience, scanning speed naturally improves because probe positioning, anatomical orientation, and measurement techniques become automatic rather than deliberate. Experienced practitioners recognize common patterns quickly and know which views will provide the most diagnostic value, allowing them to complete studies efficiently without omitting critical information. Importantly, efficiency does not mean rushing; it reflects familiarity with anatomy, pathology presentation, and machine settings. Departments often rely on experienced sonographers to maintain productivity during high-volume periods precisely because they can balance speed with diagnostic completeness.

62. How often do sonographers need continuing education?

Continuing education is a professional expectation throughout a sonographer's career. Credentialing organizations typically require ongoing continuing medical education (CME) credits to maintain certification, ensuring practitioners stay current with evolving imaging techniques, updated protocols, and new diagnostic standards. Many professionals attend workshops, conferences, or online learning programs focused on specialty imaging advancements. Continuous education not only maintains certification but also strengthens clinical confidence and opens pathways to advanced roles or specialty certifications.

63. How does technology advancement affect the sonography profession?

Ultrasound technology continues to evolve rapidly, introducing improved image resolution, 3D and 4D imaging capabilities, artificial intelligence–assisted measurements, and more portable scanning systems. These advancements expand the diagnostic capabilities of ultrasound and increase demand for skilled operators who can interpret complex imaging data effectively. Sonographers who stay current with new equipment and software updates remain highly competitive in the workforce and are often selected for specialty training opportunities within their departments.

64. What communication skills are most important in this role?

Sonographers must communicate clearly with both patients and healthcare providers. With patients, communication involves explaining procedures, addressing anxiety, and guiding positioning instructions in calm, understandable language. With physicians and clinical teams, communication requires concise technical reporting, clarification of exam findings, and prompt notification of urgent results when protocols require it. Strong communication skills improve patient cooperation, enhance workflow coordination, and contribute to accurate diagnostic outcomes.

65. How does working in emergency settings differ from scheduled outpatient imaging?

Emergency department imaging often involves unpredictable exam requests, urgent clinical indications, and patients who may be unstable, in pain, or unable to cooperate fully with positioning instructions. Sonographers in these environments must adapt quickly, perform focused exams efficiently, and maintain composure under time pressure. Outpatient imaging centers generally offer more predictable scheduling and exam pacing, though productivity expectations may still be high.

Each environment requires different workflow strategies and stress-management skills.

66. What physical self-care strategies help sonographers maintain career longevity?

Career longevity often depends on proactive physical care. Sonographers benefit from ergonomic scanning techniques, adjustable patient positioning, alternating scanning arms when possible, and regular stretching or strengthening exercises targeting shoulder and core stability. Many departments provide ergonomic training, but individual consistency in applying these techniques is essential. Professionals who prioritize body mechanics early in their careers often reduce the risk of repetitive strain injuries that can otherwise shorten time in the field.

67. How does professional reputation influence career opportunities?

Reputation plays a significant role in career mobility. Sonographers known for reliability, image quality, teamwork, and professionalism are often recommended for advanced training, leadership opportunities, or specialty assignments. Supervisors and physicians frequently rely on informal reputation when selecting staff for high-complexity exams or new technology implementation. Maintaining strong work relationships and consistent performance can therefore influence long-term career advancement as much as formal credentials.

68. What leadership opportunities exist for experienced sonographers?

Experienced professionals may transition into roles such as lead sonographer, department educator, quality assurance coordinator, or imaging supervisor. These roles involve responsibilities such as mentoring new staff, managing workflow scheduling, participating in accreditation processes, and assisting with equipment selection or protocol development. Leadership pathways allow experienced clinicians to shape departmental practices while continuing to contribute their clinical expertise.

69. How does workflow pressure influence exam quality?

High patient volumes and tight scheduling expectations can create pressure to complete exams quickly, but maintaining diagnostic quality must remain the priority. Departments that balance productivity metrics with realistic exam timing tend to produce better outcomes and reduce staff burnout. Sonographers often develop personal workflow systems—such as structured exam sequences and standardized documentation habits—that help maintain quality even during busy shifts.

70. What role does adaptability play in long-term career success?

Adaptability is one of the most valuable traits in sonography. Healthcare environments, technology platforms, clinical protocols, and patient populations change over time. Professionals who remain open to learning new techniques, adjusting workflow strategies, and pursuing additional certifications often experience greater career stability and advancement opportunities. Adaptability also supports resilience, allowing sonographers to transition between specialties or clinical settings as interests and life circumstances evolve.

71. How do sonographers handle situations when an exam reveals unexpected or serious findings?

Sonographers are often the first professionals to visually recognize abnormalities during imaging studies. When unexpected or concerning findings appear, their responsibility is to maintain professionalism, complete all required diagnostic views, and follow departmental protocols for notifying the interpreting physician or supervising clinician. They do not typically disclose diagnostic conclusions to patients, but their calm demeanor and ability to continue the exam efficiently are essential in maintaining patient confidence. Emotional intelligence is important in these moments, as patients sometimes sense that something may be wrong even when no diagnosis has been communicated.

72. How important is time management in a sonography department?

Time management directly influences both productivity and patient satisfaction. Sonographers must balance thorough image acquisition with department scheduling expectations, often working through full appointment grids that include urgent add-on cases. Effective time management involves preparing rooms in advance, organizing exam sequences efficiently, and completing documentation promptly to avoid delays that affect downstream patient flow. Departments frequently evaluate workflow efficiency metrics, making strong time-management skills a critical professional asset.

73. What is the difference between hospital-based and outpatient imaging department cultures?

Hospital-based departments often operate around the clock and manage emergency, inpatient, and surgical cases alongside scheduled exams, resulting in a faster-paced and more unpredictable environment. Outpatient imaging centers typically function on scheduled appointments with fewer emergency interruptions, offering more predictable daily pacing but still maintaining productivity expectations. Cultural differences also appear in staffing models, shift structures, and the range of exam complexity encountered. Many sonographers experience both environments during their careers and select the setting that best fits their preferred workflow style.

74. How does teamwork influence daily workflow in diagnostic imaging?

Sonography departments rely heavily on collaboration among sonographers, radiologists, cardiologists, nurses, schedulers, and transport staff. Efficient teamwork ensures patients are prepared on time, exams are prioritized appropriately, and urgent studies move quickly through the system. When communication breaks down, delays and frustration can occur across multiple departments. Professionals who consistently communicate clearly, assist colleagues during high-volume periods, and maintain cooperative working relationships often become highly valued team members.

75. What role does documentation play in the sonographer's responsibilities?

Accurate documentation is a fundamental part of the imaging process. Sonographers record measurements, annotate images, verify patient identifiers, and enter technical notes that assist interpreting physicians in generating final reports. Incomplete or inaccurate documentation can lead to repeat exams, delayed diagnoses, or billing complications. Developing consistent documentation habits early in one's career reduces errors and supports efficient departmental workflow.

76. How does certification in multiple specialties affect career flexibility?

Holding credentials in multiple sonography specialties significantly expands employment opportunities. Multi-credentialed sonographers can rotate between departments, support staffing shortages, and qualify for higher-complexity assignments. Many employers prioritize hiring professionals who can perform both general and specialty imaging because this flexibility strengthens scheduling resilience and improves departmental coverage during staffing gaps.

77. How does patient diversity influence the scanning experience?

Sonographers work with patients across all age groups, body types, mobility levels, and medical conditions. Imaging challenges can vary significantly depending on these factors, requiring adaptability in positioning techniques, probe selection, and scanning approaches. Cultural sensitivity and communication awareness are also important when interacting with diverse patient populations, ensuring procedures are explained respectfully and clearly regardless of language or background differences.

78. How do sonographers maintain professional composure during stressful situations?

Stress management skills are developed through experience, preparation, and strong workflow habits. When departments become busy or urgent cases arise, sonographers rely on structured exam routines, organized equipment setups, and clear communication to maintain control of the situation. Many professionals also develop personal stress-management strategies outside of work—exercise, adequate rest, or mindfulness practices—to sustain emotional resilience over time.

79. How does mentorship influence early-career development?

Mentorship plays a major role in the transition from student to independent practitioner. Experienced sonographers provide guidance on scanning techniques, workflow prioritization, professional communication, and department culture. New professionals who actively seek feedback and observe experienced colleagues often accelerate their skill development and confidence more quickly than those attempting to learn independently.

80. What long-term career paths exist beyond direct clinical scanning?

Beyond clinical roles, sonographers may pursue careers in education, equipment application training, research imaging, department management, or healthcare technology consulting. Some professionals work with ultrasound manufacturers as clinical specialists who train hospital staff on new equipment, while others move into academic programs to teach future sonographers. These pathways allow professionals to remain connected to the field while shifting their daily responsibilities toward leadership, innovation, or education.

81. How does workplace ergonomics influence career longevity in sonography?

Ergonomics plays a decisive role in determining how long a sonographer can comfortably remain in the profession. Repetitive scanning motions, sustained shoulder abduction, and awkward patient positioning can gradually lead to musculoskeletal injury if proper ergonomic techniques are not followed. Adjusting bed height, repositioning patients rather than overreaching, alternating scanning hands when possible, and taking brief stretching breaks during long shifts can significantly reduce long-term strain. Departments that invest in ergonomic training and adjustable equipment often see lower injury rates and longer career retention among their staff.

82. How frequently do sonographers interact with physicians during the workday?

Interaction frequency varies by department and specialty. In some settings, sonographers communicate directly with interpreting physicians multiple times per shift to clarify clinical questions or review concerning findings. In other environments, particularly high-volume outpatient centers, communication may occur primarily through structured reporting systems rather than frequent face-to-face discussions. Regardless of frequency, clear and concise communication with physicians is essential for ensuring that imaging exams answer the clinical question accurately.

83. How do sonographers stay current with advances in imaging technology?

Continuing education is required to maintain most professional credentials and serves as the primary mechanism for staying current with evolving technology. Sonographers attend workshops, complete online education modules, participate in professional conferences, and review manufacturer updates when new ultrasound systems or software upgrades are introduced. Ongoing learning ensures that professionals can take full advantage of advanced imaging capabilities and maintain high diagnostic quality.

84. What scheduling models are common in sonography departments?

Scheduling structures vary widely depending on facility type. Hospital departments often operate with rotating shifts, evening coverage, weekend rotations, and on-call responsibilities for emergency imaging needs. Outpatient imaging centers typically maintain fixed weekday schedules, though productivity expectations may still be high. Some institutions also offer flexible scheduling models, including compressed workweeks or part-time arrangements, allowing professionals to balance workload demands with personal lifestyle preferences.

85. How does workflow differ between emergency imaging and scheduled outpatient exams?

Emergency imaging requires rapid patient assessment, minimal preparation time, and adaptability to unpredictable clinical situations. Sonographers must often perform focused exams designed to answer urgent clinical questions quickly.

Scheduled outpatient exams generally allow for more structured preparation, longer appointment times, and comprehensive imaging protocols. Professionals who enjoy rapid decision-making and unpredictable workflows may prefer emergency settings, while those who value predictability may gravitate toward outpatient departments.

86. How important is adaptability in this profession?

Adaptability is one of the most valuable professional traits in diagnostic imaging. Equipment upgrades, evolving clinical protocols, changing department volumes, and rotating patient populations require sonographers to adjust their workflows frequently. Individuals who remain flexible, open to learning, and comfortable with operational changes typically navigate departmental transitions more successfully than those who strongly prefer fixed routines.

87. How does communication skill influence patient satisfaction?

Patients often judge the quality of their imaging experience based not only on technical skill but also on communication clarity and professionalism. Sonographers who clearly explain procedures, maintain calm body language, and respond compassionately to patient concerns frequently receive stronger patient satisfaction feedback. Effective communication also helps reduce patient anxiety, which can improve exam cooperation and image quality.

88. How do sonographers manage productivity expectations without sacrificing image quality?

Balancing productivity with diagnostic accuracy requires disciplined workflow habits. Preparing rooms in advance, maintaining organized supply systems, and following standardized scanning sequences allow sonographers to complete exams efficiently without omitting required imaging views. Departments that emphasize both quality assurance review and workflow efficiency training help staff maintain this balance consistently.

89. What factors contribute to long-term job satisfaction in sonography?

Long-term satisfaction often depends on a combination of supportive workplace culture, manageable productivity expectations, ergonomic equipment availability, professional growth opportunities, and scheduling flexibility. Professionals who periodically reassess their specialty alignment and work environment tend to maintain higher long-term engagement than those who remain in roles that no longer fit their personal or professional priorities.

90. How can early-career sonographers build confidence quickly?

Confidence develops through repetition, structured feedback, and progressive exposure to more complex cases. New sonographers who actively request feedback from experienced colleagues, review their own completed exams, and seek additional scanning opportunities outside of minimum requirements often build proficiency more rapidly. Over time, familiarity with normal anatomy, pathology patterns, and department workflow naturally strengthens professional confidence.

91. How does mentorship influence early career success in sonography?

Mentorship can dramatically shorten the learning curve for new sonographers. Experienced professionals provide real-time scanning tips, help troubleshoot difficult patient positioning, and explain subtle imaging findings that may not be obvious in textbooks. A supportive mentor also helps new clinicians understand department workflow, physician preferences, and communication expectations, allowing them to build confidence more quickly and avoid common early-career mistakes.

92. How does department culture affect daily work experience?

Department culture influences stress levels, teamwork quality, and long-term retention. Units that encourage collaboration, respectful communication, and shared problem-solving typically feel more sustainable than environments driven solely by productivity pressure. Even highly skilled sonographers can experience burnout in departments where teamwork is weak or expectations are unclear, making workplace culture an important factor when evaluating job opportunities.

93. How often do sonographers handle urgent or unexpected cases?

The frequency of urgent exams depends largely on the clinical setting. Hospital-based sonographers may encounter emergency add-on exams several times per shift, particularly in trauma centers or emergency departments. Outpatient centers usually experience fewer unexpected cases, though urgent physician requests can still occur. Being prepared to adjust workflow quickly is an essential part of the role.

94. What role does documentation play in sonography practice?

Accurate documentation ensures that interpreting physicians understand the clinical context of the exam and can make precise diagnostic decisions. Sonographers record technical observations, patient history details relevant to the exam, and any limitations encountered during imaging. Thorough documentation also supports quality assurance programs and helps maintain legal and regulatory compliance.

95. How does teamwork with nurses and other clinicians impact workflow?

Close collaboration with nurses, physicians, transport staff, and other imaging professionals keeps patient movement efficient and reduces delays. Clear communication about patient readiness, exam urgency, and mobility limitations allows sonographers to plan their scanning sequence effectively. Strong interdisciplinary teamwork often translates into smoother departmental operations and less daily stress.

96. How does specialty selection influence long-term career trajectory?

Choosing a specialty shapes both daily workflow and future professional opportunities. Some specialties emphasize high patient interaction and emotional conversations, while others focus more heavily on technical imaging complexity. Over time, specialty experience can lead to advanced certifications, leadership roles, education positions, or highly specialized clinical opportunities within health systems.

97. What continuing education requirements must sonographers maintain?

Most credentialing organizations require periodic continuing medical education (CME) credits to maintain active certification. These credits can be earned through professional conferences, online learning platforms, workshops, or institutional training programs. Continuing education ensures that sonographers remain current with evolving imaging techniques, safety standards, and technological advancements.

98. How do sonographers maintain consistency across high exam volumes?

Consistency comes from standardized scanning protocols, strong organizational habits, and disciplined time management. Following established imaging sequences ensures that required views are captured regardless of patient complexity or schedule pressure. Departments that implement structured quality review systems also help maintain uniform imaging standards across staff members.

99. What career advancement opportunities exist beyond routine scanning roles?

Experienced sonographers may move into lead technologist positions, departmental supervision, clinical education roles, equipment application training, research imaging programs, or quality improvement leadership. Some professionals also specialize in advanced modalities or pursue cross-training in multiple imaging specialties, expanding both responsibility and earning potential.

100. How can professionals protect long-term career sustainability in sonography?

Sustainability depends on ergonomic awareness, ongoing skill development, thoughtful specialty selection, and choosing workplaces that support reasonable productivity expectations. Professionals who proactively manage physical strain, maintain professional curiosity, and periodically reassess their work environment are more likely to remain engaged and effective throughout long careers in diagnostic imaging.

101. If I'm being completely honest with myself, should I become a Diagnostic Medical Sonographer — or would another path fit me better?

The most important question you can ask is not "Can I do this job?" but "Can I live this job, repeatedly, for years, without slowly draining the parts of myself that matter most?" Diagnostic medical sonography is often marketed as a stable, well-paying allied health profession with manageable education timelines and strong demand, all of which are true. Yet the decision to enter this field should be grounded less in the opportunity it offers and more in how the lived reality of the role aligns with your identity, temperament, physical tolerance, and long-term lifestyle goals.

Sonography is a profession built on sustained attention. During each exam, you are responsible for obtaining diagnostic-quality images while continuously adjusting probe pressure, scanning angles, machine settings, and patient positioning. The mental load is constant: observing subtle anatomical variations, identifying abnormal findings, ensuring measurements are accurate, and deciding whether additional views are required before the patient leaves the room. This level of continuous technical focus can feel deeply satisfying to individuals who enjoy precision, pattern recognition, and quiet problem-solving, but it can feel mentally exhausting to people who prefer faster-moving, task-varied environments where responsibility shifts frequently throughout the day.

The physical component of the profession is equally important to consider. Many sonographers experience repetitive shoulder strain, wrist fatigue, and back discomfort over time because scanning often requires maintaining sustained arm elevation and leaning across stretchers or exam tables for extended periods. Ergonomic training, strength conditioning, and supportive workplace practices can significantly reduce injury risk, but the physical reality of the job remains present. Individuals who thrive in sonography often accept this physical component as part of the craft, while those who struggle with repetitive strain may eventually find the work physically limiting even if they enjoy the intellectual aspects.

The emotional dimension of sonography is frequently underestimated by those considering the field. Sonographers often spend longer one-on-one time with patients than many other imaging professionals, which means they witness anxiety, uncertainty, pregnancy complications, cancer evaluations, and unexpected abnormal findings in real time. Although sonographers typically do not deliver formal diagnoses, patients frequently look to them for reassurance, interpretation, and emotional cues. Remaining calm, compassionate, and professional while maintaining diagnostic focus requires emotional steadiness and boundaries that develop with experience. For individuals who value meaningful patient interaction and quiet moments of clinical connection, this aspect of the role can feel deeply fulfilling; for those who prefer minimal emotional exposure during technical work, it may become draining over time.

Another reflection point involves pace and workflow structure. Some sonography environments—particularly emergency departments and inpatient hospitals—operate with unpredictable exam volumes, urgent add-on studies, and time pressure to move quickly between patients while maintaining image quality. Other settings, such as outpatient imaging centers or specialty clinics, may offer more predictable scheduling but still require productivity expectations that reward efficiency. Understanding which pacing environment aligns best with your personality is crucial. Some professionals thrive in the steady urgency of hospital imaging, while others perform best in controlled outpatient workflows where exams run closer to schedule.

Career sustainability also depends on how you respond to responsibility. In sonography, image acquisition is not a passive task; the interpreting physician relies heavily on the sonographer's technical judgment to ensure all necessary structures are visualized. Missing a key view can delay diagnosis or require repeat imaging, which places a meaningful level of accountability on the technologist performing the exam. Many sonographers find this responsibility motivating and professionally satisfying, while others prefer roles where diagnostic accountability is more distributed across the care team.

Financially, sonography can provide strong long-term stability, geographic flexibility, and opportunities for specialization in areas such as vascular, cardiac, obstetric, pediatric, or interventional imaging. However, income potential alone should not be the deciding factor. Sustainable career satisfaction tends to come from roles that align with how you think, how you prefer to work, how you manage physical demands, and how you handle repeated exposure to patients experiencing medical uncertainty. A slightly lower-paying role that fits your temperament can produce far greater long-term well-being than a higher-paying role that steadily depletes your physical or emotional reserves.

So the real reflection question becomes this: when you imagine yourself performing detailed imaging exams day after day—guiding patients through procedures, concentrating intensely on anatomical detail, managing the physical positioning demands of scanning, and contributing directly to the diagnostic process—does that picture feel energizing, neutral, or quietly draining? If it feels energizing or meaningfully engaging, sonography may represent strong alignment with your strengths and preferences. If it feels neutral but manageable, it may still be a viable and stable career path with the right specialty and workplace environment. But if the daily realities consistently feel misaligned with how you prefer to work or live, exploring adjacent healthcare roles that leverage your interests while better supporting your sustainability may be the wiser long-term choice.

Alignment is not about whether you are capable of succeeding in the profession. It is about whether the profession allows you to succeed **and** remain healthy, engaged, and fulfilled while doing it.

Chapter 26

What I Wish I Had Known Before Becoming a Diagnostic Medical Sonographer

Many people enter diagnostic medical sonography expecting a technical imaging role and discover, sometimes within the first few months of clinical practice, that the profession is as much about endurance, emotional awareness, and communication as it is about anatomy and equipment. If I could sit down with my younger self before the first clinical rotation, there are several things I would explain clearly — not to discourage the path, but to prepare for it.

First, I would explain that scanning is physically harder than it looks from the outside. During training, short demonstrations make the work appear smooth and effortless, yet full clinical days involve holding the arm in elevated positions for extended periods, leaning across stretchers to reach patients who cannot reposition themselves, and repeating the same motion hundreds of times per shift. The difference between a long sustainable career and an early injury often comes down to learning ergonomics early, adjusting machine positioning constantly, and protecting the shoulder even when the schedule is busy. No one emphasizes this enough at the beginning.

Second, I would explain how mentally focused the job truly is. Each exam is not simply "taking pictures"; it is a continuous diagnostic search process that requires recognizing subtle abnormalities, adjusting probe angles repeatedly, and ensuring every required anatomical view is documented before the patient leaves the room. There is very little mental autopilot available. Even routine studies require sustained concentration, and that level of constant visual decision-making can feel surprisingly draining until endurance builds over time.

Third, I would emphasize the emotional side of the profession. Sonographers are often present during some of the most vulnerable moments of patients' lives — high-risk pregnancies, emergency trauma exams, cancer evaluations, and unexpected abnormal findings. While physicians deliver final diagnoses, patients frequently read emotional cues during the exam itself, which means sonographers must balance professionalism, calm communication, and empathy even when they already suspect difficult outcomes. Learning how to remain compassionate without absorbing every emotional moment is an essential career skill that develops gradually.

I would also explain that the first job does not define the entire profession. Early positions sometimes feel overwhelming because productivity expectations are high while confidence is still developing. Many new sonographers assume that early stress reflects the entire field, when in reality different facilities, specialties, and workflow environments can feel dramatically different. Some departments move at emergency-level speed all day, while others allow longer exam times and more predictable pacing. Career satisfaction often improves significantly once individuals find the environment that matches their working style.

Another lesson I would share is that specialty training changes everything. Developing expertise in areas such as vascular imaging, echocardiography, maternal–fetal medicine, or interventional procedures can expand career mobility, increase earning potential, and make daily work more intellectually engaging. The early years of practice are an ideal time to observe which exam types feel most energizing and then intentionally pursue certification pathways that deepen those strengths.

Finally, I would remind my earlier self that confidence grows quietly. In the beginning, every exam feels like a test, every unusual finding feels intimidating, and every unfamiliar machine layout slows you down. Over time, patterns become recognizable, scanning movements become more efficient, and clinical conversations become more natural. One day you realize that what once required intense effort now feels instinctive. That transition does not happen overnight, but it does happen — and recognizing that progression helps maintain perspective during the demanding early stages of the profession.

Understanding these realities early does not make the work easier, but it makes it clearer. When people enter diagnostic medical sonography with accurate expectations about the physical demands, cognitive load, emotional exposure, and long-term specialty opportunities, they are far more likely to build careers that remain both sustainable and deeply meaningful.

1. The Physical Ergonomics Reality

Many future sonographers imagine the role as primarily technical, but few understand how physically demanding the work can become over months and years of practice. Early in training, scanning sessions are short, supervised, and scheduled with recovery time in between. Real clinical environments are different. Full shifts often involve performing exams continuously for hours, positioning patients who cannot move independently, and maintaining sustained arm elevation while applying consistent probe pressure to obtain diagnostic images. Without early ergonomic awareness, these repetitive movements can lead to shoulder strain, wrist injury, and chronic musculoskeletal issues that shorten careers.

The first lesson many experienced sonographers wish they had learned earlier is that equipment positioning matters as much as scanning technique. Adjusting bed height, bringing the patient closer rather than leaning across the stretcher, repositioning the ultrasound console frequently, and using arm support whenever possible are not minor conveniences — they are long-term career protection strategies. Small adjustments repeated throughout the day dramatically reduce cumulative strain.

Another important reality is that productivity expectations do not always allow long rest periods between exams. Departments often operate on tight schedules, and emergency add-on studies can arrive at any time. This means that ergonomic discipline must become automatic rather than optional. Sonographers who develop protective habits early often remain physically comfortable for decades, while those who "push through" poor positioning during the first few years sometimes discover injury much sooner than expected.

Strength and conditioning also play a role that training programs rarely emphasize. Maintaining shoulder stability, core strength, and posture awareness outside of work significantly improves endurance during long scanning sessions. Many veteran sonographers eventually develop personal routines that include stretching between patients, strengthening exercises at home, and deliberate recovery strategies after demanding shifts. These habits are not luxury extras — they are professional survival tools.

Understanding the physical side of the profession early changes how new sonographers approach the job. Instead of focusing only on mastering anatomy and image optimization, they begin viewing body mechanics as part of technical competence. Protecting your own physical health is not separate from patient care; it is what allows you to continue delivering high-quality imaging over many years. When ergonomics becomes part of professional identity rather than an afterthought, the long-term sustainability of the career improves dramatically.

2. The Cognitive Load Is Higher Than Expected

Many students enter sonography believing the role involves capturing predetermined image sets according to established protocols. While protocols exist, real-world scanning requires far more real-time clinical decision-making than most people anticipate. Each patient presents with different anatomy, medical histories, body habitus, and levels of mobility, requiring constant adaptation of scanning approach and image acquisition strategy. Rather than following a rigid checklist, sonographers often engage in a continuous diagnostic search process, adjusting angles, probe pressure, and imaging modes to identify structures that may not initially be visible.

This ongoing decision-making creates a level of cognitive load that can feel surprisingly intense during the first year of practice. Even routine exams demand sustained visual attention, measurement verification, and internal questioning: Have I captured every required view? Do these measurements align with clinical expectations? Is there a subtle abnormality that requires additional images? Unlike some clinical roles where tasks can become partially automated through repetition, sonography requires persistent analytical engagement throughout each examination.

The mental fatigue associated with this responsibility is rarely discussed during training. New sonographers often expect physical tiredness but are surprised by the concentration required to maintain diagnostic accuracy for an entire shift. Over time, pattern recognition improves and scanning efficiency increases, but the need for careful interpretation never disappears completely. The profession rewards attentiveness, curiosity, and a willingness to investigate unexpected findings rather than rushing through exams.

Another aspect of cognitive demand involves communication. Sonographers frequently interact with physicians, nurses, and radiologists who rely on accurate technical impressions to guide clinical decisions. While final interpretations come from interpreting physicians, the quality and completeness of the imaging dataset depend heavily on the sonographer's clinical judgment. Recognizing when to obtain additional views, when to repeat measurements, and when to escalate concerns requires both experience and confidence.

Understanding this intellectual dimension of the profession early helps new practitioners prepare mentally for the transition from student to independent scanner. The early months of practice often feel mentally exhausting not because someone lacks ability, but because the brain is rapidly building pattern recognition systems that will later operate more efficiently. Accepting that this phase is temporary allows new sonographers to view the learning curve as a normal part of professional growth rather than a personal struggle.

3. Confidence Develops Later Than You Expect

Many new sonographers assume that confidence will arrive immediately after certification, but real confidence tends to develop only after repeated exposure to varied clinical situations. The first months of independent scanning can feel uncomfortable because each patient presents unique anatomical challenges, body types, and clinical questions. Even highly capable graduates often second-guess themselves early on, wondering whether they captured every necessary image or whether subtle findings were missed. This phase is not a sign of poor preparation; it is a normal transition from supervised learning to independent clinical responsibility.

Over time, repetition builds familiarity. Structures that once required extended searching begin to appear more quickly, measurement techniques become smoother, and image optimization decisions happen almost automatically.

Experienced sonographers do not feel confident because they know everything; they feel confident because they have successfully navigated hundreds of small uncertainties and learned how to correct mistakes quickly. Recognizing that confidence is earned through experience rather than granted at graduation helps reduce the anxiety that many new professionals quietly carry during their first year.

4. Patient Communication Is as Important as Technical Skill

Many people enter sonography expecting the profession to be primarily equipment-focused, yet patient communication becomes one of the most defining aspects of daily work. Sonographers frequently interact with individuals who are anxious, uncomfortable, or worried about potential diagnoses. Explaining procedures clearly, maintaining calm body language, and responding compassionately to patient concerns often shape the patient experience as much as the technical quality of the exam.

Strong communication skills also improve scanning efficiency. When patients understand what to expect and why certain positions are necessary, they cooperate more easily, allowing images to be obtained more quickly and accurately. Over time, experienced sonographers learn that small phrases—"You're doing great," "We're almost finished," or "Let me know if that position is uncomfortable"—can significantly reduce patient tension and improve the overall flow of the exam. Technical excellence matters, but patients remember how they felt during the procedure just as strongly as the outcome.

5. Workflow Pressure Exists Even in Non-Emergency Settings

Many students believe that only emergency departments operate under time pressure, but productivity expectations exist across most sonography environments. Outpatient imaging centers often maintain tightly scheduled appointment blocks, while inpatient units require rapid responses to physician requests. Even when exams are not urgent, departments frequently track throughput metrics that encourage efficient scanning without sacrificing image quality.

Learning to balance thoroughness with efficiency becomes an essential professional skill. Experienced sonographers develop structured scanning patterns, consistent room setup habits, and mental checklists that reduce unnecessary delays. These workflow strategies allow them to maintain diagnostic quality while still meeting departmental productivity expectations. Understanding early that efficiency is a learned operational skill—not simply a personality trait—helps new practitioners focus on process improvement rather than feeling overwhelmed by early time pressures.

6. Ergonomics Can Shape the Length of Your Career

Few students fully appreciate how strongly scanning ergonomics influence long-term career sustainability. Sonographers often work in positions that require reaching across patients, holding transducers at awkward angles, or maintaining sustained shoulder elevation while concentrating on screen detail. Over time, these repetitive motions can contribute to shoulder, neck, and wrist strain if proper body positioning is not consistently practiced. Early habits matter. Adjusting bed height, repositioning equipment before beginning the exam, and using supportive arm positioning can significantly reduce cumulative stress. Experienced sonographers frequently emphasize that learning ergonomics early is not a comfort preference—it is a career protection strategy that can determine whether someone practices comfortably for decades or develops chronic musculoskeletal injuries.

7. Technology Changes Faster Than Training Programs Suggest

The imaging equipment used in clinical practice evolves continuously. Software upgrades, new transducer types, enhanced Doppler capabilities, and artificial intelligence-assisted measurement tools regularly enter departments, sometimes changing workflow expectations within months. While training programs introduce foundational scanning techniques, professional growth requires ongoing adaptation to new technologies after entering the workforce. Sonographers who remain curious, attend vendor in-services, and explore new system capabilities often become valuable departmental resources because they help colleagues transition smoothly to updated equipment. Viewing technological change as an opportunity rather than a disruption helps professionals remain adaptable and competitive throughout their careers.

8. Image Quality Often Depends on Problem-Solving, Not Just Technique

Patients rarely present with textbook anatomy. Body habitus, surgical history, medical conditions, and positioning limitations can all affect image acquisition. Successful sonographers learn to treat each exam as a problem-solving exercise, adjusting probe pressure, scanning windows, patient positioning, and machine settings until diagnostic views are achieved. This adaptive mindset distinguishes developing practitioners from highly skilled ones. The ability to troubleshoot difficult exams calmly—rather than becoming frustrated when standard approaches do not immediately work—builds professional confidence and improves diagnostic reliability. Over time, repeated exposure to challenging cases strengthens both technical creativity and decision-making speed.

9. Departments Notice Reliability as Much as Skill

Clinical environments depend heavily on consistency. Sonographers who arrive prepared, maintain organized workflows, communicate clearly with coworkers, and complete documentation accurately often become trusted team members quickly, even while still developing advanced technical skills. Reliability reduces stress for physicians, nurses, and fellow technologists because they know cases will be handled professionally from start to finish. Many supervisors quietly prioritize dependability when considering advancement opportunities such as lead technologist roles, specialty training, or cross-departmental assignments. Recognizing that professional reputation forms from daily habits—not just technical performance—encourages early attention to workflow discipline and communication.

10. Career Satisfaction Often Comes From Specialty Fit

Diagnostic medical sonography includes multiple specialties, each with different pacing, emotional exposure, and technical demands. Some professionals thrive in obstetric imaging, where long patient interactions and milestone moments are common. Others prefer vascular or cardiac environments that emphasize physiology and rapid clinical decision support. Still others enjoy outpatient abdominal imaging with predictable schedules. Discovering which specialty aligns best with personal strengths and emotional comfort can significantly influence long-term satisfaction. Many experienced sonographers encourage newcomers to explore different areas early in their careers so they can identify the environment where both skill development and daily experience feel sustainable.

11. Productivity Expectations Are Real — and Learnable

Most imaging departments track exam volumes, room utilization, and turnaround times because diagnostic imaging is closely tied to clinical decision speed. New sonographers sometimes feel pressure when they first encounter productivity benchmarks, especially if training programs emphasized technique over workflow pacing. Over time, however, efficiency becomes a learned rhythm rather than a constant stressor. Preparing rooms before patients arrive, organizing supplies consistently, and completing documentation immediately after each exam gradually reduce time pressure. Productivity is not about rushing; it is about developing repeatable systems that allow accuracy and efficiency to coexist without sacrificing patient care.

12. Communication With Physicians Improves Diagnostic Confidence

Sonographers interact frequently with interpreting physicians, particularly when unusual findings appear during an exam. Learning how to communicate observations clearly—without overstepping interpretive boundaries—strengthens collaborative trust. Experienced technologists often develop the ability to highlight concerning areas, capture additional confirmatory views, and provide concise technical impressions that help physicians interpret studies more efficiently. Strong communication skills reduce repeat exams, improve workflow continuity, and contribute to professional recognition within imaging departments.

13. Emotional Boundaries Are a Professional Skill

Because sonographers often detect abnormalities before patients receive official diagnoses, the role can involve emotionally charged moments. Maintaining empathy while protecting personal emotional well-being becomes an essential long-term skill. Professionals who develop healthy boundaries—acknowledging patient concerns while avoiding internalizing every difficult outcome—tend to sustain emotional resilience more effectively. Departments frequently provide peer support systems or informal colleague conversations that help clinicians process difficult cases. Learning to use these supports early helps prevent emotional exhaustion over time.

14. Continuing Education Is a Permanent Part of the Profession

Credential maintenance, specialty certifications, and evolving clinical standards require ongoing continuing education throughout a sonographer's career. Conferences, online modules, specialty workshops, and vendor-led training sessions help professionals maintain credentials while expanding technical expertise. Many sonographers discover that continued learning not only satisfies certification requirements but also opens opportunities for advancement into specialty roles, teaching positions, or leadership pathways within imaging departments. Viewing continuing education as a growth mechanism rather than an obligation transforms it into a long-term career advantage.

15. Your First Workplace Does Not Define Your Entire Career

New graduates sometimes assume their initial position determines their long-term trajectory, but sonography offers multiple mobility pathways. Professionals often transition between hospital systems, outpatient imaging centers, specialty labs, and mobile imaging services as their experience grows. Each environment builds different skill sets, from high-acuity emergency scanning to highly specialized vascular or cardiac imaging. Early career exploration allows individuals to identify settings that align with their preferred pace, schedule expectations, and patient populations, reinforcing the broader principle that career alignment evolves through experience rather than being decided once at graduation.

16. Equipment Familiarity Improves Both Speed and Confidence

Ultrasound systems differ widely in interface design, probe selection, measurement software, and workflow shortcuts. New sonographers sometimes feel slow simply because they are unfamiliar with a particular machine rather than lacking technical skill. Spending extra time learning preset configurations, probe optimization settings, and measurement automation tools significantly improves scanning efficiency. Over time, developing adaptability across multiple ultrasound platforms becomes a valuable professional advantage, especially for those who work in multi-site health systems or mobile imaging roles.

17. Documentation Accuracy Protects Patients and Professionals

Imaging documentation is more than administrative work; it becomes part of the permanent medical record and often guides treatment decisions. Accurate labeling of images, precise measurement entry, and clear exam notes ensure interpreting physicians receive reliable information. Documentation errors can lead to repeat exams, delayed diagnoses, or billing complications. Building the habit of reviewing measurements and labels before finalizing each exam protects both patient care and professional credibility.

18. Ergonomics Is a Career Longevity Issue

Musculoskeletal injury is one of the most common long-term risks in sonography. Reaching across stretchers, scanning with unsupported shoulders, and maintaining awkward wrist positions during long exams can gradually lead to chronic pain. Learning ergonomic scanning positions, adjusting bed height, repositioning patients when necessary, and taking brief micro-breaks between exams help reduce injury risk. Departments increasingly emphasize ergonomic education because sustaining physical health is essential for long-term career stability.

19. Department Culture Strongly Influences Job Satisfaction

Two sonography jobs with identical pay can feel dramatically different depending on workplace culture. Supportive teams, respectful physician relationships, manageable schedules, and reasonable exam volumes contribute significantly to professional satisfaction. Conversely, high turnover, chronic understaffing, and poor communication structures can create persistent stress even when compensation appears competitive. Evaluating workplace culture during interviews—asking about staffing ratios, scheduling expectations, and turnover rates—helps applicants make more informed career decisions.

20. Mentorship Accelerates Skill Development

New sonographers who work alongside experienced mentors often develop clinical confidence more quickly. Observing how senior technologists approach difficult scans, communicate with physicians, or manage complex patients provides practical learning that textbooks cannot replicate. Many professionals later become mentors themselves, creating a cycle of skill transfer that strengthens entire departments. Seeking mentorship early in a career is one of the most effective ways to build both technical competence and professional confidence.

21. Time Management Determines Daily Stress Levels

Sonography schedules can become unpredictable, especially in hospitals where emergency department and inpatient exams are added throughout the day. Developing strong time-management habits—preparing rooms efficiently, organizing supplies before the patient arrives, and completing documentation promptly after each study—helps prevent small delays from compounding into major schedule disruptions. Experienced sonographers learn to anticipate workflow bottlenecks and adjust pacing without sacrificing exam quality.

22. Communication With Physicians Requires Professional Clarity

Although sonographers do not typically provide final diagnoses, they frequently communicate directly with radiologists, cardiologists, or ordering physicians when urgent findings appear. Clear, concise communication ensures that time-sensitive information reaches the care team quickly. Learning how to describe findings using appropriate medical terminology while staying within scope of practice is an important professional skill that develops with experience.

23. Continuous Learning Is a Core Expectation of the Profession

Ultrasound technology evolves rapidly, with new imaging techniques, software upgrades, and specialty applications introduced regularly. Sonographers who pursue continuing education, additional certifications, and specialty training remain more competitive in the job market and often gain access to higher-paying roles. Lifelong learning is not optional in this field; it is a fundamental part of maintaining professional relevance.

24. Patient Anxiety Often Shapes Exam Difficulty

Many patients arrive for ultrasound exams worried about possible diagnoses, pregnancy complications, or unexplained symptoms. Anxiety can make positioning more difficult, slow exam progress, and require additional reassurance throughout the procedure. Sonographers who develop calm communication styles and patient-centered scanning approaches often complete exams more efficiently while also improving patient experience.

25. Specialty Selection Influences Long-Term Career Direction

As sonographers gain experience, many choose to specialize in areas such as vascular imaging, echocardiography, maternal-fetal medicine, or breast imaging. Each specialty offers different workflow patterns, patient populations, and career opportunities. Thoughtful specialty selection—based on personal interest, physical demands, and long-term career goals—can significantly influence professional satisfaction and advancement potential.

26. Team Coordination Improves Exam Flow

Sonographers rarely work in isolation. Coordination with nurses, physicians, transport teams, and front-desk schedulers helps maintain efficient exam flow throughout the day. When communication breaks down—patients arriving late, orders missing key information, or rooms not prepared—workflow delays quickly multiply. Strong teamwork habits, such as confirming orders in advance and communicating readiness clearly, help departments run more smoothly.

27. Understanding Clinical Indications Strengthens Image Quality

Knowing *why* an exam is being ordered helps sonographers tailor image acquisition more effectively. For example, a patient evaluated for gallstones may require slightly different image emphasis than one evaluated for liver disease. Reviewing the clinical indication before beginning each exam allows the sonographer to anticipate necessary measurements and ensures that the interpreting physician receives the most clinically relevant information.

28. Adaptability Is Essential in Hospital Settings

Inpatient and emergency department exams often require scanning patients who cannot easily reposition, hold their breath, or tolerate long exam times. Sonographers frequently adapt scanning techniques—modifying probe angles, adjusting patient positioning creatively, or capturing images quickly when patient stability is limited. Flexibility under these circumstances becomes a defining professional skill.

29. Quality Control Protects Diagnostic Reliability

Routine quality assurance processes, including equipment calibration, image review audits, and protocol standardization, ensure consistent diagnostic reliability across departments. Sonographers who participate actively in quality initiatives help maintain departmental credibility and reduce the need for repeat exams caused by incomplete or technically inadequate studies.

30. Career Growth Often Comes Through Skill Diversification

Expanding into multiple specialties, learning new imaging protocols, or developing expertise in advanced procedures can open pathways to leadership roles, education positions, or supervisory responsibilities. Diversifying technical skills not only improves job security but also increases flexibility when exploring new employment opportunities or geographic relocation.

31. Documentation Accuracy Matters as Much as Image Quality

Precise documentation—including measurements, patient positioning notes, technical limitations, and procedural observations—ensures that interpreting physicians understand the context of the images obtained. Incomplete documentation can lead to misinterpretation, repeat exams, or delays in clinical decision-making, making thorough recordkeeping a critical professional responsibility.

32. Workload Fluctuations Require Mental Endurance

Some days move steadily according to schedule, while others shift rapidly with emergency add-ons, inpatient requests, and unexpected complex exams. Sonographers learn to maintain mental stamina during unpredictable workload spikes, staying attentive to detail even when exam volume is high or schedules fall behind.

33. Patient Comfort Directly Affects Exam Success

Positioning discomfort, anxiety, or pain can limit a patient's ability to cooperate during scanning. Taking a few extra moments to adjust pillows, explain breathing instructions, or reassure nervous patients often results in clearer images and shorter overall exam times. Patient-centered scanning frequently improves both technical outcomes and patient satisfaction.

34. Equipment Maintenance Awareness Prevents Workflow Disruptions

Although biomedical departments handle major repairs, sonographers are often the first to notice early signs of equipment malfunction—loose probes, inconsistent image brightness, or software glitches. Prompt reporting of minor issues helps prevent larger failures that could delay patient care or cancel scheduled exams.

35. Emotional Boundaries Help Sustain Long-Term Career Health

Repeated exposure to patients facing serious diagnoses, pregnancy complications, or chronic illness can create emotional fatigue over time. Sonographers who develop healthy professional boundaries—balancing compassion with emotional self-protection—are more likely to maintain long-term resilience and avoid burnout.

36. Efficient Room Preparation Reduces Daily Stress

Preparing rooms with stocked gel, linens, cleaning supplies, and probe covers before patient arrival prevents unnecessary interruptions during exams. Small organizational habits accumulated over time significantly reduce workflow stress and allow sonographers to focus more fully on patient care and image acquisition.

37. Continuous Learning Is a Core Professional Expectation

Advancements in imaging technology, evolving clinical guidelines, and new specialty certifications require sonographers to remain engaged in ongoing education. Continuing education courses, professional conferences, and credential expansion not only maintain licensure requirements but also support professional growth and adaptability.

38. Interpersonal Skills Influence Workplace Reputation

Technical skill alone does not define professional success. Reliability, respectful communication with coworkers, willingness to assist teammates, and responsiveness to physician requests all shape a sonographer's reputation within a department. Strong interpersonal professionalism often leads to better scheduling flexibility and career advancement opportunities.

39. Ergonomic Technique Protects Career Longevity

Proper probe grip, machine positioning, and scanning posture help reduce the risk of repetitive strain injuries that affect many imaging professionals. Departments increasingly emphasize ergonomic training because early technique habits strongly influence whether sonographers remain physically comfortable throughout their careers.

40. Reflection Helps Guide Career Alignment Decisions

Periodic reflection—evaluating workload preferences, specialty interests, scheduling tolerance, and emotional demands—helps sonographers determine whether their current role continues to align with long-term personal and professional goals. Career satisfaction often improves when individuals make intentional adjustments rather than remaining in roles that gradually drain energy.

41. Strong Time Management Prevents Exam Backlogs

Sonographers often work within tightly scheduled appointment blocks where even small delays can ripple through the entire day. Efficient preparation, quick transitions between patients, and disciplined adherence to scanning protocols help maintain workflow stability while still preserving exam quality. Time management becomes a learned professional rhythm rather than a rushed reaction.

42. Communication With Interpreting Physicians Improves Diagnostic Accuracy

Radiologists, cardiologists, and other interpreting providers rely on sonographers to communicate technical challenges, unusual patient positioning issues, or suspected abnormal findings. Clear verbal or electronic communication ensures physicians understand the context of the exam, reducing the risk of incomplete diagnostic interpretation.

43. Specialty Certification Expands Career Options

Obtaining additional credentials in vascular, cardiac, obstetric, pediatric, or breast imaging can open access to higher-paying roles, specialty departments, or supervisory opportunities. Many sonographers build careers by gradually stacking certifications that align with their professional interests and departmental needs.

44. Night and Weekend Coverage Requires Lifestyle Adaptability

Hospitals often operate ultrasound services 24 hours a day, meaning sonographers may rotate through night shifts, weekend schedules, or on-call responsibilities. Individuals who adapt well to irregular schedules may find increased earning potential, while those who prefer consistent routines may gravitate toward outpatient imaging environments.

45. Confidence Builds Gradually Through Case Exposure

New sonographers often feel uncertain when first encountering complex anatomy or abnormal findings. Over time, repeated exposure to varied patient cases builds visual recognition skills and scanning confidence. Experience gradually transforms hesitation into calm, methodical decision-making during challenging exams.

46. Professional Networking Supports Career Mobility

Connections made through clinical training sites, professional associations, conferences, and workplace teams often lead to future job opportunities. Many imaging professionals discover that career mobility frequently depends as much on professional relationships as on formal job postings.

47. Productivity Expectations Differ Between Settings

Hospital imaging departments, outpatient centers, and specialty clinics operate under different productivity benchmarks. Understanding these differences helps sonographers choose work environments that match their preferred pace, patient interaction level, and scheduling expectations.

48. Patient Education Is Part of the Clinical Role

Patients frequently arrive with limited understanding of what ultrasound exams involve. Sonographers often provide brief procedural explanations, answer common questions, and clarify what patients can expect during the exam. Effective patient education improves cooperation, reduces anxiety, and enhances overall care experiences.

49. Team Trust Develops Through Consistent Performance

Departments quickly learn which sonographers consistently produce high-quality studies, communicate clearly, and handle unexpected workload surges effectively. Over time, dependable performance builds trust with physicians and colleagues, often leading to expanded responsibilities or leadership opportunities.

50. Career Satisfaction Often Depends on Specialty Fit

Some sonographers thrive in high-acuity hospital environments with unpredictable workloads, while others prefer structured outpatient imaging schedules. Identifying which clinical pace, patient population, and workflow environment aligns best with personal strengths can significantly influence long-term career satisfaction.

51. Continuous Learning Is a Core Expectation in Imaging

Diagnostic medical sonography is not a static profession. Ultrasound systems evolve regularly, incorporating new imaging modes, enhanced Doppler capabilities, artificial-intelligence-assisted measurements, and specialty-specific software updates that change how examinations are performed. Sonographers who view graduation or initial certification as the endpoint of learning often find themselves struggling to keep pace within only a few years. Continuing education courses, specialty credentialing, professional conferences, and department-based training sessions allow sonographers to refine technique, expand diagnostic awareness, and maintain clinical confidence as new technologies emerge. Beyond technical advantages, ongoing education signals professionalism to employers and often becomes a prerequisite for advancement into specialty, lead, or educational roles. The sonographers who build long careers in imaging rarely stop learning; instead, they treat professional development as a routine part of maintaining clinical excellence rather than an occasional requirement.

52. Ergonomic Awareness Protects Long-Term Career Longevity

Musculoskeletal injury is one of the most significant occupational risks in diagnostic sonography. Repetitive shoulder abduction, prolonged static arm positioning, scanning across stretchers, and pushing heavy ultrasound equipment contribute to chronic strain that can shorten careers if not actively managed. Ergonomic awareness is therefore not a minor workplace consideration but a foundational professional skill. Proper patient positioning, adjusting bed height before beginning an exam, bringing equipment closer to the body, alternating scanning arms when possible, and scheduling short recovery intervals between lengthy exams all help reduce cumulative physical stress. Many experienced sonographers emphasize that the scanning habits developed during the first five years of practice often determine whether an individual remains comfortable in the field twenty years later. Investing attention in ergonomics early is one of the most practical long-term career protection strategies available in imaging.

53. Workflow Flexibility Helps Departments Handle Surges

Unlike highly predictable outpatient scheduling environments, hospital-based imaging departments frequently experience sudden surges in exam volume driven by emergency department arrivals, inpatient clinical changes, or add-on procedures requested throughout the day. Sonographers who demonstrate workflow flexibility—adjusting priorities quickly, assisting colleagues during peak volume periods, and remaining calm during schedule disruptions—become invaluable operational contributors. Flexibility does not mean working without structure; it means maintaining procedural discipline while adapting to shifting clinical demands. Departments that function smoothly during high-volume periods typically rely on imaging professionals who understand that healthcare delivery is dynamic rather than linear. Professionals who learn to operate comfortably within this fluid environment often experience stronger performance evaluations and greater opportunities for expanded responsibility over time.

54. Documentation Accuracy Is as Important as Image Quality

Producing technically excellent images is only part of the diagnostic process. Measurements, annotations, exam notes, patient identifiers, and procedural documentation must be entered with equal precision to ensure the interpreting physician receives a complete clinical record. Inaccurate labeling, missing measurements, or incomplete documentation can delay interpretation, require repeat imaging, or contribute to clinical misunderstanding. Many departments maintain strict documentation protocols precisely because imaging studies become permanent components of the patient's medical record and may influence treatment decisions long after the examination is completed. Sonographers who develop consistent documentation habits early in their careers reduce error risk, support physician workflow efficiency, and strengthen patient safety. In practice, thorough documentation becomes a professional signature—an indicator that the imaging professional values diagnostic completeness as much as technical performance.

55. Interpersonal Skills Improve Patient Cooperation

Diagnostic imaging frequently places sonographers in direct contact with patients who may be anxious, in pain, or uncertain about the medical concerns prompting the examination. Calm communication, clear procedural explanations, respectful physical assistance, and attentive listening often determine whether patients are able to remain still long enough for optimal image acquisition. Even technically skilled sonographers may struggle to obtain diagnostic images if patients are uncomfortable or fearful during the exam. Effective interpersonal interaction therefore functions as a technical performance multiplier: when patients feel informed and supported, they are more likely to cooperate with breathing instructions, positioning requests, and exam duration requirements. Over time, sonographers who consistently demonstrate strong patient-centered communication skills often become trusted departmental professionals who are requested for more complex or sensitive examinations.

56. Strong Anatomy Knowledge Drives Diagnostic Accuracy

Ultrasound imaging is fundamentally dependent on the sonographer's ability to understand three-dimensional anatomy while working with two-dimensional imaging planes. Unlike imaging modalities that rely more heavily on automated acquisition, ultrasound requires the operator to locate structures manually, adjust probe orientation continuously, and recognize subtle variations in normal and abnormal anatomy in real time. This means anatomy knowledge is not simply an academic prerequisite; it is a daily working tool that determines exam quality. Sonographers who maintain strong anatomical awareness can identify structures more efficiently, adjust scanning windows when visualization becomes challenging, and recognize early signs of pathology that may require additional views. Over time, anatomy mastery becomes one of the key differences between technically competent sonographers and highly trusted imaging professionals whose exams consistently support confident physician interpretation.

57. Time Management Directly Affects Department Performance

Imaging departments often operate under productivity expectations that balance patient access with diagnostic quality. Sonographers who manage exam time effectively—preparing rooms in advance, reviewing patient history before scanning, organizing workflow between cases, and maintaining steady scanning pace without rushing—help departments remain on schedule while preserving care standards. Poor time management, by contrast, can create cascading delays that affect physician interpretation timelines, patient satisfaction, and overall operational efficiency. Effective time management does not mean performing exams as quickly as possible; rather, it involves developing a consistent rhythm that allows each exam to be completed thoroughly while respecting departmental flow. Professionals who demonstrate dependable pacing often become valued team members because their workflow reliability contributes to smoother department operations.

58. Communication With Physicians Improves Diagnostic Collaboration

Although sonographers typically do not issue final diagnostic interpretations, their communication with interpreting physicians plays a critical role in ensuring that imaging studies capture clinically relevant information. When sonographers clearly communicate unusual findings, technical limitations, or patient-specific concerns, physicians can tailor interpretation or request additional views that strengthen diagnostic confidence. This collaborative communication may occur through direct conversation, documentation notes, or departmental messaging systems depending on the setting. Sonographers who develop professional, concise communication habits help create a diagnostic partnership that improves patient care outcomes. Over time, physicians often come to rely heavily on sonographers whose clinical observations demonstrate consistency and sound judgment.

59. Adaptability Is Essential When Equipment Varies Across Facilities

Not all ultrasound systems operate identically. Differences in machine manufacturers, software interfaces, probe selection, preset configurations, and measurement workflows can require rapid adaptation when sonographers change departments, accept travel assignments, or transition between healthcare systems. Professionals who become comfortable learning new equipment quickly maintain productivity more easily across varied environments. Adaptability includes understanding imaging principles well enough to translate scanning techniques regardless of the machine being used, rather than relying exclusively on memorized button sequences from a single system. Sonographers who cultivate this equipment flexibility often experience smoother onboarding transitions and broader employment opportunities across different clinical settings.

60. Professional Reputation Builds Career Mobility Over Time

In many healthcare environments, employment opportunities often circulate through professional networks, departmental recommendations, and informal reputation signals long before formal job postings appear. Sonographers who consistently demonstrate reliability, teamwork, patient-centered care, and technical competence gradually build professional reputations that travel with them throughout their careers. Supervisors may recommend them for specialty training, colleagues may alert them to openings in desirable departments, and recruiters may prioritize candidates known for strong performance. Reputation is rarely established through one exceptional moment; it develops through repeated demonstrations of professionalism across everyday clinical interactions. Over the long term, a positive professional reputation becomes one of the most powerful drivers of career mobility within the imaging field.

61. Ergonomic Awareness Protects Long-Term Career Longevity

Musculoskeletal injury is one of the most significant occupational risks in diagnostic medical sonography. Repetitive scanning motions, sustained shoulder elevation, leaning across patients, and awkward wrist positioning can gradually lead to strain injuries affecting the shoulder, neck, wrist, and lower back. Sonographers who prioritize ergonomic positioning—adjusting bed height, positioning the patient correctly before scanning, keeping the scanning arm close to the body, and using supportive equipment when available—significantly reduce the likelihood of long-term injury. Departments increasingly emphasize ergonomic education because experienced sonographers lost to preventable injury represent both a workforce loss and a personal career disruption. Professionals who treat ergonomics as a daily discipline rather than an occasional adjustment are more likely to maintain career longevity and physical sustainability.

62. Patient History Review Improves Scan Efficiency and Diagnostic Value

Reviewing the patient's clinical history prior to beginning an exam allows sonographers to tailor scanning strategy toward the most clinically relevant findings. Understanding the reason for the study, prior imaging results, laboratory abnormalities, or known diagnoses helps guide probe selection, imaging depth, measurement priorities, and the selection of additional views when necessary. Sonographers who consistently review patient history before scanning often complete exams more efficiently because they avoid unnecessary imaging sequences and focus on answering the clinical question driving the study. This preparation also strengthens communication with physicians, as sonographers can contextualize findings within the patient's broader clinical picture.

63. Continuing Education Keeps Skills Aligned With Advancing Technology

Ultrasound technology continues to evolve, introducing improved imaging resolution, new Doppler capabilities, advanced 3D/4D imaging techniques, and specialized procedural applications. Sonographers who engage regularly in continuing education—through conferences, online coursework, specialty credential preparation, or departmental training—remain better equipped to adapt to emerging clinical demands. Continuing education is not only a certification maintenance requirement; it is also a professional investment that expands employment opportunities, supports specialty transitions, and enhances diagnostic confidence. Over time, professionals who remain engaged in learning often become informal departmental resources when new technologies are introduced.

64. Department Culture Strongly Influences Job Satisfaction

Two sonography positions with identical compensation and workload expectations can feel dramatically different depending on departmental culture. Supportive teams that communicate clearly, distribute workload fairly, and respect scheduling boundaries often create environments where sonographers feel professionally valued. In contrast, departments characterized by chronic understaffing, poor communication, or inconsistent leadership support may contribute to faster burnout even when pay is competitive. Evaluating workplace culture during interviews—observing staff interactions, asking about turnover rates, and learning how scheduling conflicts are handled—can provide early insight into long-term job satisfaction potential. Alignment with team culture frequently influences career sustainability as much as technical job responsibilities.

65. Emotional Intelligence Helps Navigate Sensitive Patient Encounters

Sonographers frequently interact with patients undergoing emotionally sensitive examinations, including pregnancy assessments, cancer evaluations, trauma imaging, and chronic disease monitoring. Emotional intelligence—the ability to recognize patient anxiety, communicate calmly, maintain professional boundaries, and respond appropriately to emotional reactions—plays a critical role in patient experience. While sonographers must avoid providing diagnostic interpretations, they still serve as primary patient contacts during imaging procedures, making their communication style highly impactful. Professionals who develop strong emotional awareness often create more reassuring patient experiences while also protecting their own emotional well-being through healthy professional boundaries.

66. Workflow Adaptability Improves Performance Across Clinical Settings

Diagnostic medical sonographers work in a wide range of clinical environments, including hospitals, outpatient imaging centers, emergency departments, physician offices, mobile imaging services, and specialty clinics. Each setting operates at a different pace, with distinct workflow expectations, documentation systems, and patient populations. Professionals who demonstrate workflow adaptability—quickly learning scheduling systems, adjusting scanning pace to match departmental demand, and understanding how to prioritize urgent exams—tend to integrate more smoothly into new teams. Adaptability becomes particularly valuable when transitioning between roles or accepting per-diem or travel assignments, where orientation periods may be brief and performance expectations immediate.

67. Documentation Accuracy Protects Both Patient Care and Professional Liability

Accurate exam documentation ensures that interpreting physicians receive clear information regarding imaging findings, exam limitations, and any technical challenges encountered during the procedure. Proper documentation includes labeling images correctly, recording measurements precisely, noting patient positioning, and documenting any deviations from standard protocol. Incomplete or inaccurate documentation can delay diagnosis, require repeat exams, or create medico-legal vulnerabilities. Sonographers who develop disciplined documentation habits early in their careers reduce error risk and build professional credibility within their departments.

68. Professional Certifications Expand Career Flexibility and Advancement Opportunities

Many sonographers begin their careers with a single specialty credential, but additional certifications—such as vascular, cardiac, breast, or pediatric imaging—can significantly broaden employment opportunities. Multi-credentialed sonographers often qualify for float roles across multiple departments, specialty pay differentials, supervisory tracks, and advanced clinical responsibilities. Certification expansion also provides career resilience, allowing professionals to pivot specialties if departmental demand shifts or personal interests evolve over time. Investing in additional credentials is often one of the most direct ways to increase long-term earning potential and job mobility.

69. Productivity Metrics Influence Departmental Expectations

Healthcare organizations frequently track productivity metrics such as exams completed per shift, average exam duration, patient wait times, and departmental throughput. While quality of imaging remains the primary responsibility, sonographers must also learn to balance thorough scanning with time efficiency to meet operational expectations. Understanding how productivity metrics function helps professionals pace their workflow appropriately, anticipate scheduling pressures, and communicate realistically with supervisors when exam complexity affects throughput. Departments that openly communicate productivity expectations tend to support more transparent workload management.

70. Interprofessional Collaboration Strengthens Diagnostic Accuracy

Sonographers rarely work in isolation. Daily collaboration occurs with radiologists, cardiologists, obstetricians, vascular surgeons, nurses, technologists, and administrative staff. Effective communication ensures that imaging requests are appropriate, exam priorities are clear, and critical findings are escalated promptly. Sonographers who build strong interprofessional relationships often find that workflow becomes smoother, communication barriers decrease, and patient care coordination improves. Collaboration also supports professional learning, as interaction with physicians and specialty clinicians deepens clinical understanding beyond imaging technique alone.

71. Emotional Intelligence Shapes the Patient Experience

Technical accuracy is only part of effective sonography practice. Patients often arrive anxious, uncomfortable, or uncertain about what their imaging exam might reveal, and the sonographer becomes the person guiding them through that moment. Emotional intelligence—the ability to read emotional cues, respond with calm reassurance, and maintain professional composure during sensitive encounters—greatly influences patient experience. Sonographers who develop strong interpersonal awareness are often trusted more quickly by patients, which improves cooperation during positioning and scanning and ultimately contributes to better image quality.

72. Equipment Familiarity Improves Efficiency and Reduces Stress

Although ultrasound systems operate on similar principles, each manufacturer and facility configuration introduces unique controls, presets, and workflow settings. Sonographers who invest time early in each new assignment learning machine shortcuts, preset adjustments, and probe optimization features often work more efficiently and experience less performance stress during busy shifts. Familiarity with equipment also reduces troubleshooting time when technical issues arise, allowing exams to continue smoothly without unnecessary delays.

73. Time Management Skills Prevent Daily Backlogs

Sonography schedules can shift rapidly when emergency add-on exams, inpatient requests, or complex cases interrupt planned workflows. Effective time management involves balancing thorough imaging with practical pacing, communicating anticipated delays to scheduling teams, and preparing rooms quickly between exams. Sonographers who master time awareness—without rushing patient care—help departments maintain flow while reducing overtime pressure on staff. Over time, strong time management becomes one of the most valued operational skills within imaging departments.

74. Continuing Education Sustains Long-Term Career Growth

Healthcare technology, imaging protocols, and certification standards evolve continuously. Continuing education ensures that sonographers remain current with emerging scanning techniques, updated clinical guidelines, and regulatory requirements tied to credential maintenance. Participation in conferences, online learning modules, specialty workshops, and professional organizations not only fulfills certification requirements but also exposes professionals to new subspecialties and leadership opportunities. Lifelong learning supports both career advancement and long-term professional relevance.

75. Self-Care Practices Protect Career Longevity

The physical and emotional demands of sonography can accumulate over time if recovery habits are neglected. Repetitive scanning movements, emotionally difficult patient encounters, and productivity pressure all contribute to fatigue if left unmanaged. Consistent stretching routines, ergonomic awareness, regular physical conditioning, and mental decompression practices after intense clinical days help sustain career longevity. Sonographers who treat recovery as a professional responsibility—not a luxury—often remain healthier and more satisfied in the field across many years of practice.

76. Communication With Physicians Requires Precision and Confidence

Sonographers frequently interact with interpreting physicians to clarify exam indications, confirm imaging priorities, or communicate urgent findings that require immediate review. Clear, concise clinical communication helps ensure that physicians receive the information necessary to interpret images accurately and make timely care decisions. Confidence in speaking about imaging observations—while remaining within scope—strengthens collaboration and professional credibility within the care team.

77. Workflow Adaptability Is Essential in Hospital Settings

Unlike highly predictable outpatient imaging centers, hospital environments require sonographers to pivot quickly between scheduled exams, emergency requests, and inpatient studies across multiple floors. Adaptability allows professionals to maintain composure when priorities shift without warning. Those who remain flexible and solution-focused during workflow disruptions often become invaluable team members because they help departments maintain continuity even during high-volume periods.

78. Documentation Accuracy Protects Clinical Decisions

Measurements, annotations, exam notes, and patient identifiers must be recorded with absolute precision because diagnostic interpretations rely heavily on the accuracy of captured data. Even small documentation errors can lead to confusion, repeat imaging, or delayed care decisions. Sonographers who build consistent documentation habits early—double-checking identifiers, measurement labels, and technical notes—reduce clinical risk and strengthen the reliability of diagnostic workflows.

79. Professional Reputation Develops Faster Than Many Expect

Within healthcare systems, reputations spread quickly through informal professional networks. Sonographers known for reliability, teamwork, and consistent imaging quality often find themselves offered specialty training, leadership roles, or preferred scheduling opportunities sooner than peers who struggle with consistency. Early attention to professionalism, punctuality, and collaborative behavior can significantly influence long-term career opportunities.

80. Specialty Diversification Expands Career Flexibility

Developing competence across multiple sonography specialties—such as vascular, obstetrics, abdominal, or cardiac imaging—broadens employment options and improves long-term job security. Facilities experiencing staffing shortages often prioritize professionals who can float between exam types, allowing them to support multiple departments. Over time, cross-specialty experience also creates pathways into education, management, or advanced clinical leadership roles.

81. Patient Positioning Skills Directly Influence Image Quality

Even the most advanced imaging equipment cannot compensate for poor patient positioning. Understanding how body alignment, breathing instructions, and probe angle adjustments affect visualization is central to producing diagnostic-quality images. Experienced sonographers develop positioning strategies that account for patient discomfort, injury limitations, and body habitus while still obtaining necessary views efficiently.

82. Mentorship Accelerates Early Career Development

New sonographers who seek mentorship from experienced colleagues often progress more quickly in technical confidence, workflow efficiency, and specialty readiness. Mentors provide practical shortcuts, ergonomic advice, and insight into department culture that cannot be learned from textbooks alone. Facilities that cultivate strong mentorship environments frequently see better staff retention and stronger clinical skill development among new hires.

83. Ethical Responsibility Includes Maintaining Patient Privacy

Imaging professionals regularly encounter sensitive medical information, emotional patient conversations, and personal clinical histories. Maintaining strict patient confidentiality, both in documentation and casual workplace conversation, is a professional obligation tied to regulatory compliance and ethical care standards. Consistent privacy awareness protects patients and strengthens trust in healthcare systems.

84. Stress Recognition Prevents Burnout Escalation

High productivity expectations, emotionally difficult cases, and physical strain can gradually elevate stress levels without immediate recognition. Sonographers who learn to identify early signs of fatigue—such as irritability, persistent soreness, or decreased concentration—can take proactive steps to adjust workload patterns, request ergonomic support, or strengthen recovery routines before burnout intensifies.

85. Career Satisfaction Often Depends on Environment Fit

Two sonographers performing identical exams may experience dramatically different job satisfaction depending on leadership support, scheduling flexibility, team culture, and productivity expectations. Choosing work environments that align with personal pacing preferences, communication style, and lifestyle priorities often has a greater long-term impact on satisfaction than salary differences alone.

86. Clinical Pattern Recognition Develops Through Repetition and Reflection

One of the most important professional transitions in sonography occurs when scanning moves from purely mechanical image acquisition to meaningful clinical pattern recognition. Early in a career, sonographers focus heavily on probe positioning, measurement accuracy, and following protocol step-by-step. With experience, however, the brain begins to recognize subtle visual patterns—unexpected shadowing, unusual vessel flow characteristics, asymmetry in organ appearance, or anatomical distortions that suggest evolving pathology. This ability does not come from memorization alone; it develops through repeated exposure, reviewing physician reports after completed exams, and mentally connecting imaging findings with eventual diagnoses. Sonographers who intentionally study outcomes after their exams gradually build a deeper diagnostic awareness that improves exam completeness, reduces missed structures, and strengthens their clinical value to interpreting physicians.

87. Workflow Anticipation Reduces Department Bottlenecks

Highly effective sonographers do more than complete individual exams; they learn to anticipate how their workflow interacts with the broader imaging department. Recognizing when emergency department demand is rising, when inpatient transport delays may affect scheduling, or when high-complexity exams will require longer scan times allows professionals to adjust pacing proactively. Preparing rooms early, coordinating with scheduling teams, or communicating anticipated delays helps prevent cascading bottlenecks that affect the entire department. Over time, departments often rely heavily on sonographers who demonstrate this systems-level awareness because they contribute not only technical skill but also operational stability.

88. Professional Boundaries Protect Emotional Sustainability

Because sonographers spend extended one-on-one time with patients, they often become recipients of deeply personal conversations involving illness, pregnancy anxiety, chronic disease, or unexpected diagnoses. Compassionate listening is essential, yet maintaining professional emotional boundaries is equally important for long-term sustainability. Sonographers who attempt to carry every patient's emotional burden home may gradually experience compassion fatigue, whereas those who learn to provide empathy while preserving emotional separation are better able to sustain long careers without psychological exhaustion. Structured decompression routines—such as brief reflection breaks between difficult exams, peer discussion, or end-of-shift mental resets—can significantly improve emotional resilience.

89. Technology Comfort Level Influences Career Advancement

Modern ultrasound platforms continue to evolve with advanced imaging modes, automation tools, AI-assisted measurement systems, and integration with electronic medical records. Sonographers who remain curious about new technology, volunteer for equipment training, and develop comfort troubleshooting machine performance often position themselves for leadership roles such as super-user status, department educator positions, or equipment selection committees. Technical curiosity therefore becomes more than a personal interest; it can directly influence long-term advancement opportunities and professional recognition within imaging departments.

90. Long-Term Career Satisfaction Often Comes From Role Design, Not Role Title

Many professionals initially assume that career fulfillment will come from promotions or job title changes, yet long-term satisfaction in sonography frequently depends more on how a role is structured than what it is called. Schedule flexibility, exam mix variety, supportive leadership, ergonomic resources, and realistic productivity expectations often determine daily well-being more than formal rank. Sonographers who intentionally evaluate these environmental factors when choosing positions—and who advocate for adjustments when misalignment appears—are more likely to sustain both performance and personal satisfaction throughout their careers.

91. Building Cross-Department Relationships Improves Daily Workflow

Imaging departments operate in constant coordination with emergency physicians, inpatient units, outpatient clinics, transport teams, and scheduling staff. Sonographers who cultivate positive working relationships across departments often experience smoother patient flow, quicker communication during urgent cases, and stronger support when unexpected workflow challenges arise. Professional courtesy, responsiveness, and collaborative problem-solving gradually create informal professional networks that make demanding clinical environments far easier to navigate.

92. Ergonomic Awareness Must Be Practiced Daily, Not Occasionally

Musculoskeletal injury remains one of the most significant occupational risks in sonography. Proper scanning posture, equipment height adjustment, shoulder positioning, and patient bed alignment must become automatic habits rather than occasional corrections. Small daily ergonomic decisions accumulate over years; consistently practicing protective positioning can significantly reduce long-term shoulder, neck, and wrist injuries that otherwise shorten careers. Departments increasingly recognize this risk and may provide ergonomic training, but individual awareness remains the most powerful protective factor.

93. Documentation Narratives Help Interpreting Physicians Understand Context

While images are central to diagnostic interpretation, concise technical notes written by sonographers often provide important procedural context—patient positioning challenges, limited visualization due to pain, or technical adjustments made during scanning. These short documentation narratives help interpreting physicians understand exam limitations and avoid misinterpretation of technically restricted views. Clear documentation therefore contributes directly to diagnostic accuracy and patient safety.

94. Mentoring Students Strengthens Personal Clinical Mastery

Teaching students or new hires frequently deepens a sonographer's own expertise because explaining scanning techniques requires organizing knowledge in a structured way. Mentors often refine their own positioning strategies, exam sequencing, and troubleshooting skills as they demonstrate procedures step-by-step. Over time, many experienced professionals discover that mentoring not only supports workforce development but also renews their own professional engagement and pride in the craft.

95. Career Longevity Is Strongly Influenced by Recovery Habits Outside Work

Sustaining a multi-decade career in sonography depends heavily on what professionals do outside the imaging suite. Strength training, flexibility routines, sleep consistency, hydration, and stress-management practices all play a meaningful role in preserving physical capacity and mental clarity. Sonographers who treat recovery as part of their professional toolkit—rather than an afterthought—often maintain higher performance levels and greater job satisfaction across long careers.

96. A New Specialty Can Save Your Career Without You Leaving Sonography

I used to think feeling bored or restless meant I was falling out of love with the profession, but a lot of the time it meant I had outgrown my current lane. Sonography has enough branches—vascular, cardiac, maternal-fetal medicine, pediatrics, breast imaging, interventional guidance—that you can change your day-to-day reality without starting over. Learning a new specialty brings back challenge, reactivates curiosity, and can honestly make you feel like yourself again at work. If you ever hit that "I can't do this forever" feeling, consider whether you need a new career—or just a new specialty.

97. Your Reputation Travels Faster Than Your Resume

I wish someone had told me that the way you show up on ordinary days matters more than one impressive exam. People notice who stays calm, who is prepared, who owns mistakes, who helps without being asked, and who keeps the room steady when things get tense. That reputation quietly shapes everything: who gets offered specialty training, who gets first pick of schedules, who gets trusted with harder cases, and who gets promoted. You don't have to be perfect, but you do have to be consistent.

98. Money Grows Through Strategy, Not Just Time

Early on, I assumed pay would rise automatically with experience, but a lot of sonographers stall because they never think strategically about income. Compensation can change dramatically based on specialty, certifications, shift differentials, overtime patterns, and geography. If you want stronger long-term stability, you have to periodically evaluate your market value and make aligned moves—adding a credential that fits you, moving into a specialty you can sustain, or changing settings when your current one caps your growth. Raises are nice, but career design is what changes your financial future.

99. The Meaning You Get From the Work Will Change Over Time

In the beginning, meaning comes from mastering the machine, getting faster, capturing perfect views, and surviving the steep learning curve. Later, the "why" often shifts. You may find meaning in how you reassure patients, how you mentor new techs, how you improve workflow, or how you catch something subtle that changes a diagnosis. If you expect meaning to feel the same forever, you'll think you're losing something when you're actually evolving.

100. Sometimes You Don't Hate Sonography, You Hate Your Department

I wish I had learned earlier to separate the profession from the environment. Productivity pressure, leadership culture, staffing, scheduling, and the way a department treats people can make a job feel unbearable even if you still love the actual work. Before you decide you're "done," ask whether you're done with sonography—or done with this setting. A different environment can completely change your nervous system, your energy, and your ability to stay in the field long-term.

101. The Real Question Isn't "Can I Do This?" It's "Can I Sustain This?"

Most people can learn the technical skills if they work hard enough, but sustainability is a different test. Sonography asks for long stretches of focus, hands-on precision, constant patient interaction, and the quiet responsibility of producing images that drive medical decisions. If that rhythm energizes you more often than it drains you—and the physical and emotional realities feel manageable with time—this path may fit you beautifully. If the repetitive strain, pace, or emotional load consistently feels like it's taking more than it gives, another role might fit your life better. The win is choosing the career whose daily reality matches who you are, not just what you're capable of.

Chapter 27

The Field Isn't Changing, It's Transforming

Walk into an imaging department five or ten years from now and it will feel noticeably different from the one you trained in. The machines will be sleeker and more portable. Ultrasound will show up at the bedside in more specialties, more units, and more moments of clinical decision-making. Software will quietly assist with measurements and standardization. Physicians will lean on imaging support during procedures that used to be done "by feel." And in many pathways, ultrasound will become the first test ordered, not the backup.

This chapter is not about technology replacing sonographers. It is about technology amplifying sonographers. The future of ultrasound is not a story of substitution; it is a story of expansion. Ultrasound is becoming the stethoscope of modern medicine, and sonographers are becoming the interpreters of that language—people who translate motion, flow, anatomy, and subtle change into information a care team can act on. Let's step into that future together.

Part 1 — Technology That's Already Changing the Game

1. AI-Enhanced Imaging

Think of AI as a co-pilot, not a replacement. It will not scan patients for you, and it will not diagnose. What it will do is reduce friction and increase consistency. AI tools are already being developed and integrated to suggest probe angle improvements for standard views, assist with Doppler placement, auto-label and organize images, highlight regions that may warrant closer attention, support measurement consistency, and reduce common documentation errors. The biggest practical value is endurance—AI does not get tired, distracted, or rushed at the end of a long shift. Sonographers who understand how to use AI responsibly will become the people departments rely on for quality improvement, training, and workflow refinement.

2. Point-of-Care Ultrasound (POCUS)

POCUS is rapidly expanding across emergency medicine, critical care, anesthesia, hospital medicine, OB triage, cardiology, sports medicine, and even prehospital settings. It is easy to hear that growth and assume it threatens sonography. In practice, it often does the opposite. POCUS creates more ultrasound, not less. It increases demand for training, quality oversight, confirmatory diagnostic studies, and clear protocols for when a bedside scan is enough and when it is not. POCUS does not replace sonographers; it depends on them. In many systems, sonographers become the stabilizing force that keeps bedside ultrasound accurate, consistent, and clinically safe.

3. Handheld Ultrasound Devices

Handheld systems are becoming smaller, more capable, and more affordable. As these devices spread into primary care offices, urgent care sites, ambulatory clinics, and rural settings, the need for expertise grows alongside access. Handheld ultrasound democratizes imaging; it does not automatically ensure quality. That is where sonographers become essential as trainers, protocol builders, quality champions, and the professionals who can step in when a quick look turns into a high-stakes diagnostic question. The more ultrasound becomes "everywhere," the more the healthcare system needs people who truly understand how to do it well.

4. Elastography and Advanced Tissue Imaging

Elastography and other advanced applications are raising the complexity ceiling of the profession. These tools support assessments in liver fibrosis, thyroid disease, oncology, breast imaging, and musculoskeletal care, and they demand careful protocol mastery, anatomical judgment, and consistent measurements that stand up under clinical scrutiny. As advanced capabilities expand, the role becomes less about "capturing an image" and more about executing a sophisticated diagnostic study that clinicians rely on for decisions. That is elevation, not erosion.

Part 2 — The Role of the Sonographer Is Expanding

5. Sonographers as Clinical Decision Partners

Sonographers are not diagnosticians, but they increasingly function as high-skill collaborators who influence what happens next. In many settings, you will be expected to recognize when additional views are needed, identify when an exam is drifting off protocol, escalate urgent concerns through the right channels, and communicate clearly so interpretation and care planning move quickly. Over time, your judgment becomes part of the department's reliability—one of the reasons physicians trust imaging as a decision-making tool rather than a passive service.

6. Sonographers in Procedural Medicine

Ultrasound guidance continues to expand across procedures such as biopsies, line placement, thoracentesis, paracentesis, abscess drainage, nerve blocks, and injections. As procedure volume grows, so does the need for professionals who can obtain consistent visualization, anticipate workflow needs, and maintain patient calm while a team is focused on precision. The more procedural medicine uses ultrasound, the more teams rely on sonographers who understand both imaging quality and clinical pacing.

7. Tele-Ultrasound and Remote Support

Remote guidance is not science fiction. It is a practical tool for improving access, especially in rural hospitals and underserved regions where specialized ultrasound expertise may not be available on-site. Tele-ultrasound models can support real-time second opinions, remote mentoring for newer staff, and better access to specialists. This is not primarily a job-loss story; it is a reach story. It allows expertise to travel farther than the clinician can, which can expand both impact and career options.

8. Sonographer-Led Specialty Clinics

In some markets, sonographer-forward models are already emerging in vascular labs, fibrosis clinics, vein centers, thyroid programs, and high-throughput prenatal assessment units. These environments rely on advanced protocols, strong quality systems, and sonographer expertise functioning at the front edge of diagnostic pathways. When done well, they create clearer triage, faster access, and more consistent studies, and they open doors to leadership, specialization, and workflow ownership.

Part 3 — Career Paths of the Future

9. The Rise of the Advanced Sonographer Role

Many systems are moving toward more stratified imaging roles: entry-level, experienced, and advanced practice-style positions that carry responsibilities beyond scanning. These roles may include protocol oversight, quality assurance, staff training, POCUS education support, workflow redesign, research collaboration, and sometimes structured preliminary communication processes within policy limits. The early adopters in these pathways are often the people who later become leads, educators, and department anchors.

10. Hybrid Roles in Clinical Technology

As ultrasound becomes more integrated with software and AI, hybrid roles will expand: clinical workflow specialists, product testers, application specialists, clinical AI trainers, ultrasound data and quality analysts, and imaging consultants. Sonographers who can speak both languages—the real clinical workflow and the technical toolset—will be valuable in hospitals, academic centers, and industry environments. Healthcare technology companies consistently seek clinicians who understand what actually happens in exam rooms and what breaks when software is designed without bedside reality.

11. Travel Sonography 2.0

Travel work is also shifting. In many markets, demand is trending toward specialized, short-term, high-need staffing; rural access initiatives; crisis coverage; and roles tied to expertise such as vascular, cardiac, high-risk OB, and procedural support. The earning potential rises when you are able to fill gaps that fewer professionals can cover, and the future of travel will increasingly reward specialization, adaptability, and clinical maturity.

12. Research Sonographers Becoming Essential

Large clinical trials, new imaging protocols, AI algorithm development, and precision medicine require consistent scanning, strong documentation, and reproducible technique. Research sonographers often become the bridge between protocol design and real-world execution. If you enjoy structure, consistency, and clinical curiosity, this pathway can be both stable and highly influential.

Part 4 — What This Means for You

13. Your Skills Will Be More Valuable, Not Less

Demand for ultrasound is growing, and the human parts of the job remain irreplaceable. AI cannot position patients safely, earn trust from anxious people, adapt to pain or fear in real time, make micro-adjustments based on anatomy and body habitus, or provide the calm, steady presence patients remember. Those aren't side details—they are core components of quality.

14. The Best Sonographers Will Blend Art and Science

The future belongs to sonographers who remain grounded in anatomy, measurements, Doppler fundamentals, and protocol discipline while also learning to use new tools responsibly. The strongest professionals will be the ones who can adapt without losing empathy, who can learn software without becoming mechanical, and who can keep the patient at the center even as technology becomes more sophisticated.

15. You Can Build a Future-Proof Career

If you stay teachable, keep your skills current, protect your body, remain emotionally grounded, and maintain intellectual curiosity, you will remain indispensable for decades. The "future-proof" sonographer is not the one who knows everything today; it is the one who keeps evolving without compromising quality or humanity.

The Bottom Line

The future of Diagnostic Medical Sonography is not one of replacement. It is one of expansion, elevation, and innovation. Sonographers will collaborate more, teach more, specialize more, guide more, and influence more of the pathways that determine care. Ultrasound is becoming a central language of modern medicine, and sonographers are the professionals who speak it fluently when it matters most.

Chapter 28

Professional Development Roadmap

The Journey Begins Before the Classroom

No one becomes a sonographer overnight. There's no single path, elevator, shortcut, or magic bullet.

What there *is* — is a **roadmap**. A real, workable, doable progression.

This chapter walks you through:

- what to do first,
- what to do next,
- how to grow,
- how to specialize,
- how to advance, and
- how to build a career that doesn't just pay the bills but genuinely *fits* you.

Whether you're 18, 28, 48, or 68 — this roadmap applies.

PHASE 1 — EXPLORATION

"Do I Actually Want to Be a Sonographer?"**

1. Learn What the Field Really Involves

Most people think ultrasound = babies.

This book has now shown you the truth: it's anatomy, pathology, precision, pressure, fear, hope, and human stories.

You should explore:

- DITLs (like the ones in this book)
- Interviews with sonographers
- Real ultrasound cases on YouTube
- Program open houses
- Job shadowing
- Professional organizations

This is the curiosity phase.

Follow your spark.

2. Assess Your Strengths and Fit

Ask yourself:

- Do I like anatomy?
- Can I stay calm in stressful situations?
- Do I enjoy interacting closely with people?

- Am I detail-oriented?
- Can I stay compassionate when others are scared?

If the answer is "mostly yes," you're in the right place.

PHASE 2 — FOUNDATIONS

Prerequisites, Planning, and Picking the Right Program**

3. Complete Your Prerequisites

Most programs require:

- Anatomy & Physiology I & II
- College-level math
- Physics (sometimes specific to radiation sciences)
- Medical terminology
- Communication or English
- Possibly psychology

Get good grades — competitive programs *do* care.

4. Choose Your Pathway

Options include:

- **Accredited Sonography Certificate Program** (often 12–20 months)
- **Associate Degree** in Diagnostic Medical Sonography
- **Bachelor's Degree** (less common but expanding)
- **Cross-training** if you're already in imaging

The best choice?

The one that's CAAHEP accredited.

5. Apply to Multiple Programs

Because programs are competitive, it's smart to apply to several.

You may need:

- letters of recommendation
- a personal statement
- proof of observation hours
- transcripts
- interviews

Treat applications like a job search — professionally and proactively.

PHASE 3 — EDUCATION

School, Simulation, and the Art of Not Panicking**

6. Survive — and Thrive — in the Didactic Phase

Expect classes in:

- sonographic physics
- cross-sectional anatomy
- abdominal scanning
- OB/GYN
- vascular

- pathology
- instrumentation
- patient care

This phase is heavy.

You're learning an entire language of sound waves.

7. Clinical Rotations: Where You Become a Sonographer

This is the heart of your training.

You'll rotate through:

- hospitals
- outpatient clinics
- OB practices
- vascular labs
- NICUs
- ER departments

You'll learn:

- how to talk to patients
- how to document accurately
- how to manage fear in the room
- how to scan in real, imperfect conditions
- what specialty you actually love

Your confidence will grow one scan at a time.

8. Build Relationships With Mentors

Mentors are the bridge between "student" and "hireable."

They'll teach you:

- tips for difficult body types
- shortcuts for finding tough anatomy
- how to handle demanding physicians
- how to manage bad news
- how to survive stressful days

Keep every good mentor close.

You'll thank yourself later.

PHASE 4 — CERTIFICATION

Your Credentials Become Your Passport

9. Sit for Registry Exams (ARDMS, CCI, or ARRT)

You earn credentials like:

- **RDMS** — Abdomen, OB/GYN
- **RVT** — Vascular
- **RDCS** — Cardiac
- **RMSKS** — Musculoskeletal

These letters open doors.

Hospitals trust them.

Managers prefer them.

Specialties require them.

Plan ahead — registry exams require serious study.

10. Become Job-Ready

Create:

- a polished resume
- a standout cover letter
- a list of references
- a clean, short skills summary
- a list of your preferred specialties

You're not just looking for *a* job — you're looking for the right fit.

PHASE 5 — EARLY CAREER

Your First Job, Your First Wins, Your First Hard Days**

11. Learn How to Survive the First Year

Your first year is about:

- building speed
- building confidence
- learning workflow
- navigating personalities
- refining communication
- trusting your instincts

Your technique will improve dramatically with repetition — and patience.

12. Specialize (or Don't Yet — That's Okay Too)

Early in your career, you may explore:

- OB
- vascular
- general
- cardiac
- MSK
- transplant
- IR
- oncology
- pediatrics

You don't have to know on day one.

Your specialty might find *you*.

13. Protect Your Body

Start early:

- adjust your ergonomics
- stretch daily
- strengthen your core
- report equipment issues
- use proper stool and table heights

Burnout is physical *and* emotional.

Guard both.

PHASE 6 — GROWTH & MASTERy

Choosing Your Signature Specialty and Building a Future**

14. Become the Go-To in Your Department

This happens naturally when you:

- scan consistently well
- handle difficult cases calmly
- communicate professionally
- support your coworkers
- maintain reliability

People will start requesting you by name.

That's when you know:

you're becoming *that sonographer.*

15. Consider Advanced Paths

Once you feel grounded, you can grow into:

Advanced Clinical Specialist

Specialize deeply in OB, MFM, vascular, cardiac, or oncology.

Lead Sonographer / Supervisor

Run the team. Manage workflow. Train new hires.

Education & Instruction

Teach the next generation — clinical instructor, program faculty.

Travel Sonography

High pay, mobility, short-term contracts.

Research Sonography

Clinical trials, academic hospitals, novel imaging techniques.

Industry Roles

Applications specialist, product trainer, equipment consultant.

Master's or Bachelor's Completion routes

If leadership or teaching is a long-term plan.

16. Build a Long, Sustainable Career

The sonographers who last decades share three habits:

- They protect their mental health
- They protect their physical health
- They stay curious and never stop learning

Longevity isn't luck — it's cultivation.

The Bottom Line

Becoming a Diagnostic Medical Sonographer isn't a sprint or a gamble.

It's a roadmap, and you now have the whole thing in front of you.

Follow it with:

- intention
- curiosity
- humility
- courage
- compassion

And this field will give back more than you can imagine.

Chapter 29
PACES™ & CARESET™

PACES™ & CARESET™ in Diagnostic Medical Sonography — Why This Career Fits Some People Beautifully and Drains Others Quietly

The work of a Diagnostic Medical Sonographer is far more than operating an ultrasound machine. It requires sustained concentration, physical endurance, emotional composure, patient-facing communication, and precise clinical judgment performed in real time. Some professionals thrive in this environment for decades; others discover that the pace, physical demands, or workflow constraints quietly erode their energy over time. Understanding that difference begins with alignment.

Two frameworks used throughout the ScrubTales™ series help readers evaluate that alignment: **PACES™** and **CARESET™**. PACES™ focuses on the individual—how your wiring, preparation, and life context interact with the profession. CARESET™ focuses on the environment—how workplace conditions shape sustainability, performance, and long-term satisfaction. Together, they help explain why the same role can feel energizing to one person and exhausting to another.

PACES™ — Understanding Personal Alignment in Sonography

Personality

Diagnostic medical sonography rewards individuals who are detail-oriented, patient, observant, and comfortable working in focused clinical environments where concentration must remain steady for extended periods. Sonographers often interact with patients during vulnerable moments—prenatal imaging, cardiac studies, emergency diagnostics—so emotional steadiness and calm interpersonal presence play an important role in daily success. Those who prefer rapid task switching or highly social, constantly changing workflows may find the repetitive precision of imaging more taxing over time.

Aptitude

The role demands strong visual-spatial reasoning, anatomical recognition, pattern identification, and technical equipment mastery. Sonographers must recognize subtle differences between normal and abnormal findings while simultaneously adjusting probe positioning, depth, gain, and Doppler settings in real time. Comfort with technology, anatomy, and measurement accuracy supports both performance and professional confidence.

Constraints

Work schedules, shift structures, ergonomic strain, family responsibilities, and geographic mobility all influence how sustainable the career feels. Some imaging departments operate with call requirements, extended standing periods, or high patient volumes that may not align with every individual's physical needs or life circumstances. Recognizing personal constraints early helps professionals select work settings that better match their long-term lifestyle goals.

Experience

Previous healthcare exposure, clinical rotations, and early mentorship strongly influence how quickly new sonographers adapt to workflow demands. Hands-on clinical learning environments that emphasize structured scanning protocols, communication with radiologists, and exposure to varied patient populations accelerate professional confidence and reduce early-career stress.

Situation

Life stage, financial pressures, commuting demands, and local job-market dynamics all shape career experience. A setting that feels ideal early in a career may require adjustment later as professional priorities, family needs, or leadership aspirations evolve. Evaluating the "situation" dimension ensures that career decisions reflect real-world context rather than idealized assumptions about the profession.

CARESET™ — Understanding Environmental Alignment in Sonography

While PACES™ explains the personal side of alignment, **CARESET™** describes the environmental conditions that determine whether professionals can perform at their best over time.

Culture

Departmental culture influences everything from teamwork and communication to workload expectations and psychological safety. Imaging departments that promote collaboration with radiologists, nurses, and physicians—and that support respectful patient interactions—tend to foster higher retention and stronger professional satisfaction.

Autonomy

The degree of decision-making authority granted to sonographers varies by institution. Some departments allow experienced technologists meaningful clinical discretion in protocol adjustments and workflow prioritization, while others maintain tightly structured processes. Alignment between autonomy level and individual preference significantly affects job satisfaction.

Resources

Equipment quality, staffing levels, ergonomic supports, continuing-education funding, and administrative responsiveness all shape daily work experience. Adequate resources reduce physical strain, scanning backlogs, and burnout risk, while insufficient resources can gradually transform a technically rewarding profession into a physically demanding one.

Expectations

Productivity metrics, exam turnaround times, call requirements, and patient-volume expectations determine workload intensity. Clear, realistic expectations enable professionals to maintain quality imaging while protecting long-term sustainability; unrealistic expectations often lead to fatigue, repetitive-strain injuries, and reduced engagement.

Structure, Environment, Team

Workflow organization, physical department layout, leadership accessibility, and team cohesion directly influence performance. Departments with coordinated scheduling, supportive supervisors, and collaborative interdepartmental communication create environments where sonographers can focus on clinical excellence rather than operational friction.

Why PACES™ and CARESET™ Matter in Sonography

A career in diagnostic medical sonography is not defined only by technical skill. Long-term success depends on the interaction between who you are (**PACES™**) and where you work (**CARESET™**). When both align, the profession can provide decades of meaningful, intellectually engaging, and patient-centered work. When they do not, even highly capable professionals may find themselves quietly depleted. Understanding these frameworks early allows you to choose training paths, specialties, and workplaces that support not only competence—but sustainability.

Chapter 30

Mistakes Don't Define You, but Ignoring Them Will

Every sonographer enjoys talking about the compelling pathology they identified, the difficult cases they solved, the beautiful fetal scans they captured, the vascular exams they helped clarify, and the trauma moments where they remained calm under pressure. Ask them about mistakes, however, and the stories usually come quietly. Most experienced sonographers carry entire libraries of early-career missteps that shaped how they practice today. This chapter brings those quiet lessons into the light so new sonographers do not have to learn everything the hard way. The reality is simple: you will make mistakes. It is part of becoming skilled. What matters is learning to recognize patterns early so they do not repeat.

Pitfall 1 — Letting Nerves Take Over the Exam

New sonographers often feel their hands tense and their thoughts scatter when the pressure of performing in front of a preceptor or anxious patient rises. This happens because you want to impress your team, reassure the patient, and avoid missing pathology all at the same time. Pressure can briefly hijack performance. The solution is simple but powerful: pause before beginning, take a slow breath, mentally visualize the anatomy, and quietly outline your scanning plan. If you lose orientation, reposition, reset, and continue. Confidence is not the absence of nerves; it is continuing to scan effectively even while feeling them.

Pitfall 2 — Overfocusing on Images While Ignoring the Patient

Early in training, many sonographers become so focused on obtaining perfect images that they unintentionally disconnect from the person on the table. Patients may feel dismissed or unseen, even when the scan is technically excellent. Make brief eye contact before and after the exam, explain what you are doing, and periodically check on the patient's comfort. The most respected sonographers maintain technical precision while preserving human connection.

Pitfall 3 — Rushing the Exam

Speed feels urgent in busy departments, especially when emergency cases or add-on exams begin stacking up. However, rushing early in your career increases the likelihood of missed anatomy or incomplete documentation. Follow the progression that experienced professionals understand well: accuracy first, consistency second, and speed third. Speed arrives naturally once the first two are mastered.

Pitfall 4 — Not Asking for Help When You Are Stuck

Many new graduates hesitate to ask for assistance because they fear appearing inexperienced. In reality, asking for a second set of eyes demonstrates professionalism and patient-safety awareness. A simple request such as, “Could you take a quick look with me to make sure I’m not missing anything?” builds trust and prevents small uncertainties from becoming larger issues.

Pitfall 5 — Mislabeling or Under-Labeling Images

Fatigue, rushing, and inconsistent habits can lead to labeling errors that create confusion during interpretation. Establish a consistent mental checklist for orientation, labeling, and annotation. Slow down briefly to confirm accuracy; the clarity of your images determines how effectively the clinical team can act on your findings.

Pitfall 6 — Incomplete Documentation

Sometimes a sonographer recognizes an abnormality but fails to capture enough supporting images or measurements to justify the finding. When uncertain, over-document rather than under-document. Capture orthogonal views, obtain Doppler evaluation when appropriate, and include cine loops for complex areas. Documentation is not only a technical task; it directly supports patient safety.

Pitfall 7 — Skipping Protocol Steps

As experience grows, familiarity can create the temptation to skip steps during seemingly routine exams. Protocols exist to protect both patient and practitioner. Even on busy days, following structured exam sequences ensures subtle pathology is not missed in blind spots created by shortcuts.

Pitfall 8 — Letting Emotion Guide Communication

Patients may ask difficult questions about findings that cannot be discussed until the interpreting physician reviews the study. Emotional situations can make it tempting to reassure or speculate. The safest response is compassionate neutrality, such as, "Your physician will review everything with you very soon," while continuing to provide calm support during the exam.

Pitfall 9 — Physical Burnout from Poor Ergonomics

Reaching too far, twisting the torso, or scanning at improper bed heights can gradually produce shoulder, wrist, or back strain. Adjust the bed and stool before every exam, maintain neutral wrist positioning, use core strength rather than isolated arm movement, and take brief stretching breaks between patients. Protecting your body is essential for sustaining a long career.

Pitfall 10 — Not Trusting Your Clinical Instincts

New sonographers sometimes dismiss their intuition when an image "doesn't look right," assuming the concern reflects inexperience. Instead, capture additional images, adjust angles, obtain Doppler when appropriate, or request a second opinion. Clinical instincts strengthen with use; honoring them improves diagnostic confidence.

Pitfall 11 — Communication Hesitation with Physicians

When a radiologist or cardiologist requests additional views, uncertainty can make newer technologists freeze rather than clarify expectations. Professional collaboration sounds simple: "Of course—would you like a Doppler sweep or a closer margin view?" Clear communication strengthens teamwork and reduces repeat scanning.

Pitfall 12 — Taking Every Critique Personally

Early-career professionals often interpret feedback as a personal failure. In reality, healthcare environments are fast-paced, and most colleagues are focused on patient care rather than judging individual performance. Treat feedback as technical guidance rather than personal evaluation, and improvement accelerates quickly.

Specialty-Specific Pitfalls

Different ultrasound specialties introduce their own learning curves. In obstetrics and gynecology, challenges may include recognizing adnexal masses, accurately measuring cervical length, or managing emotionally difficult no-heartbeat exams. In vascular imaging, incorrect Doppler angles or incomplete vessel tracking can affect interpretation. Cardiac imaging requires careful avoidance of artifact misinterpretation and consistent ventricular measurements. Interventional radiology support demands precise needle visualization and continuous communication during procedures. Neonatal imaging requires careful pressure control and awareness of delicate anatomy, while oncology imaging demands careful measurement tracking and emotional resilience when working with long-term patients.

How to Become a Safe Sonographer

Professional growth follows consistent habits: ask questions when uncertain, never conceal near-misses, document carefully, follow established protocols, remain humble, and maintain compassion for both patients and colleagues. These habits transform early mistakes into long-term mastery.

The Bottom Line

Every sonographer makes mistakes. With awareness, humility, curiosity, discipline, and compassion, those mistakes become the foundation of clinical wisdom. The most respected technologists are not perfect—they are attentive, present, and committed to learning from every scan.

Chapter 31

Financial Landscape™ — The Long Payback

Choosing a healthcare career is not only an identity decision; it is also a long-term financial commitment. Education costs, certification requirements, relocation decisions, shift structures, and specialty pathways all shape the economic trajectory of a Diagnostic Medical Sonographer. Understanding the financial realities early allows you to make decisions that protect both your professional stability and your personal life.

Many students enter sonography programs focused primarily on program acceptance, clinical placement, and certification success. What often receives less attention is the full economic picture that unfolds during the first ten years of practice. Income growth, specialty selection, geographic flexibility, overtime opportunities, and loan repayment strategies can dramatically alter long-term financial outcomes. Two professionals graduating from the same program in the same year may experience entirely different financial realities depending on how intentionally they navigate those variables.

Education Investment and Early Career Return

The cost of sonography education varies widely depending on the pathway chosen. Certificate programs often require lower tuition but may have highly competitive admission standards. Associate and bachelor's degree programs generally carry higher costs but may provide broader academic foundations and expanded clinical exposure. Regardless of the pathway, most graduates enter the workforce with some level of educational debt, and the early years of employment often become a balancing act between establishing clinical competence and stabilizing personal finances.

Early career salaries in diagnostic medical sonography typically provide a solid starting point relative to many healthcare roles requiring similar training durations. However, the perception that healthcare automatically guarantees financial comfort can be misleading. The first years after graduation frequently involve relocation decisions, certification exam costs, licensing fees in certain states, continuing education requirements, and the purchase of professional essentials such as uniforms, credentialing renewals, and specialty exam preparation materials. Understanding these additional expenses prevents unrealistic expectations about immediate disposable income.

The Compounding Effect of Specialty Selection

One of the most powerful financial variables in sonography is specialty focus. While general sonography roles provide stable employment opportunities, advanced specialties such as vascular imaging, echocardiography, pediatric sonography, and high-risk obstetrics often command higher compensation over time due to the complexity of the exams and the smaller supply of trained professionals. Professionals who strategically pursue additional certifications early in their careers often see long-term income advantages that compound over decades.

Specialty selection also influences scheduling patterns. Some specialties involve more call responsibilities, emergency coverage, or high-acuity inpatient work, which can increase total compensation through differential pay. Others offer more predictable outpatient schedules with fewer call demands but potentially lower overall earnings. Financial planning therefore becomes less about chasing the highest hourly rate and more about choosing the structure that aligns with long-term lifestyle sustainability.

Geographic Mobility as a Financial Lever

Geography plays a major role in sonographer compensation. High-demand metropolitan areas, rapidly growing suburban regions, and underserved rural healthcare systems frequently offer signing bonuses, relocation assistance, or higher base salaries to attract experienced professionals. Cost-of-living differences must always be evaluated alongside salary increases, but geographic flexibility can significantly accelerate early financial progress, particularly during the first five years of practice when income growth tends to occur most rapidly.

Some professionals intentionally spend several years working in higher-demand regions to reduce educational debt more quickly before transitioning to locations that better match long-term lifestyle preferences. Others prioritize remaining near family or support networks and pursue specialty certifications instead to increase earning potential without relocating. Both strategies can be effective when approached intentionally rather than reactively.

Loan Repayment Strategy and Financial Stability

Educational loans influence career flexibility more than many students initially realize. Monthly repayment obligations can shape job selection decisions, overtime willingness, and even specialty choices. Developing a structured repayment plan early—whether through accelerated repayment, income-driven plans, or employer-sponsored assistance programs—reduces long-term financial stress and allows greater freedom when considering future career moves.

Some healthcare systems, academic institutions, and underserved-area employers offer loan repayment incentives or tuition assistance for advanced certifications. These programs can significantly alter long-term financial outcomes but often require service commitments that should be evaluated carefully before acceptance. Understanding the full terms of repayment assistance programs ensures that short-term financial relief does not unintentionally restrict future mobility.

Income Growth Over the First Decade

Unlike some professions where compensation remains relatively static, sonography income often increases meaningfully with experience, specialty credentials, and demonstrated clinical reliability. The first two years typically focus on skill consolidation and departmental integration. Years three through five often bring certification expansion, cross-training opportunities, and eligibility for differential pay or advanced scheduling options. By the second half of the first decade, many professionals move into senior sonographer, lead technologist, specialty coordinator, or supervisory roles that provide both financial and professional advancement.

Understanding this progression prevents early-career discouragement. Initial salaries represent the starting point of the trajectory, not the long-term ceiling. Strategic certification timing, willingness to cross-train, and consistent performance reliability significantly influence how quickly professionals move along the compensation curve.

The Hidden Financial Impact of Burnout

Financial planning is not only about income generation; it is also about career longevity. Repetitive strain injuries, chronic scheduling fatigue, and unmanaged stress can shorten careers prematurely, reducing lifetime earnings more dramatically than any single salary negotiation. Ergonomic awareness, specialty diversification, and thoughtful workload selection protect both physical health and long-term financial stability. Professionals who remain healthy and engaged in the field for decades often achieve far greater cumulative earnings than those who maximize short-term income while neglecting sustainability.

Financial Alignment as a Career Strategy

The goal of financial planning in sonography is not simply to earn more; it is to create a career structure that supports stability, flexibility, and long-term professional satisfaction. When education investment, specialty development, geographic choices, and repayment strategies are aligned intentionally, the profession offers strong long-term economic potential. When decisions are made reactively—chasing the highest hourly rate without considering sustainability—financial stress can persist despite competitive salaries.

The Long Payback is not only about loans; it is about understanding how early career decisions ripple forward across decades. Sonographers who approach the financial dimension of their careers with the same analytical mindset they bring to imaging studies often find themselves better positioned for both professional longevity and personal financial confidence.

Chapter 32

Building a Resume That Gets Diagnostic Medical Sonographers Hired

Landing a position as a Diagnostic Medical Sonographer requires more than strong scanning skills. Hiring managers often review dozens—sometimes hundreds—of applications for a single opening, and the résumé becomes the first demonstration of your professionalism, clarity of thought, and readiness to step into patient care. A well-constructed résumé does not simply list where you trained; it communicates what you can do safely, independently, and consistently from day one. The goal of this chapter is to help you build a résumé that clearly shows employers that you are prepared, reliable, and capable of contributing immediately.

Start With a Clean, Professional Structure

Healthcare hiring leaders spend very little time on their first résumé review. Clarity matters more than design complexity. Your résumé should typically be one page for new graduates and early-career professionals, expanding to two pages only after several years of specialized experience. Use clear headings, consistent spacing, and a readable font. Avoid graphics, unusual formatting, or dense blocks of text that make scanning difficult. A hiring manager should be able to understand your qualifications within the first fifteen seconds.

At the top of the résumé, include your full name, credentials (such as RDMS, RVT, RDCS, or registry-eligible status), phone number, professional email address, and city/state location. This section should be clean and prominent, as it establishes immediate credibility.

Lead With a Clinical Skills Summary

Many applicants begin with education, but in clinical hiring, employers are primarily asking one question: "What exams can this person safely perform?" A short clinical skills summary directly under your contact information helps answer that question immediately. This section should list your scanning competencies, specialties, and equipment familiarity. For example, include areas such as abdominal ultrasound, OB/GYN, vascular Doppler, echocardiography views, small parts imaging, or pediatric exposure if applicable. Mention familiarity with PACS systems, reporting software, or EHR platforms if you have used them during clinical training.

The purpose of this section is not to exaggerate expertise but to clearly communicate operational readiness. Even registry-eligible candidates can demonstrate readiness by listing exam types performed during clinical rotations.

Present Education and Certifications Clearly

Your education section should include the name of your sonography program, degree or certificate earned, graduation date, and any honors received. Immediately beneath this, list certifications or registry status. If you have passed credentialing exams such as ARDMS, CCI, or ARRT, list the full credential and year obtained. If you are registry-eligible and scheduled to test, state this clearly (for example, "ARDMS registry-eligible; exam scheduled July 2026"). Hiring managers value clarity because credential timelines often affect hiring decisions.

Highlight Clinical Rotation Experience as Professional Experience

For new graduates, clinical rotations function as professional experience and should be presented with the same seriousness as employment. List each clinical site, location, and rotation dates, followed by concise bullet points describing exam volume exposure, specialties encountered, and responsibilities. Instead of writing "Completed clinical rotation," describe the scope of experience: "Performed abdominal, pelvic, and small-parts exams under supervision; assisted with vascular Doppler studies; participated in ER add-on imaging workflow; gained experience in portable bedside scanning." These descriptions help employers understand how quickly you may transition into independent practice.

Quantify Whenever Possible

Numbers make résumés stronger because they demonstrate exposure and readiness. When possible, include approximate exam counts, specialties performed, or workflow participation. For example: "Participated in high-volume outpatient clinic performing approximately 15–20 abdominal exams per day" or "Assisted in vascular lab performing carotid, venous reflux, and arterial Doppler studies." Quantification helps hiring leaders estimate orientation needs and training timelines.

Include Technical Competencies and Equipment Familiarity

Diagnostic imaging departments often operate with multiple ultrasound platforms, and familiarity with common systems can strengthen candidacy. If you trained on specific machines or software platforms, list them in a technical skills section. This may include ultrasound systems (for example, GE, Philips, Siemens, Mindray), reporting platforms, or PACS systems. This section reassures employers that onboarding may be smoother.

Demonstrate Professional Reliability and Team Skills

Healthcare hiring decisions are not based solely on technical skill. Reliability, professionalism, and communication matter deeply. If you have prior healthcare experience, customer service experience, or roles demonstrating responsibility, briefly include them—especially if they highlight teamwork, patient communication, or schedule reliability. Departments often prioritize candidates who show professionalism and coachability, even when technical experience is still developing.

Avoid Common Resume Mistakes

Several résumé habits unintentionally weaken strong candidates. Avoid listing unrelated personal details, overly long objective statements, or vague phrases such as "hardworking" or "team player" without supporting examples. Proofread carefully; spelling or formatting errors create an impression of inattention to detail, which is particularly concerning in imaging professions where precision matters. Also avoid overly decorative formatting or multi-column templates that may not scan well in applicant tracking systems.

Prepare a Focused Cover Letter to Accompany the Resume

While some systems treat cover letters as optional, a short, thoughtful cover letter can differentiate you. Use it to express interest in the specific department, highlight your clinical strengths, and demonstrate enthusiasm for learning. Keep it concise—one page or less—and connect your training experiences to the environment you are applying for, such as inpatient, outpatient, vascular lab, or cardiac imaging settings.

Update the Resume as You Grow

A résumé should evolve continuously. After your first job, update exam competencies, specialty training, continuing education, and certifications. Over time, your résumé shifts from education-centered to experience-centered, reflecting increasing independence and specialization. Maintaining an updated résumé ensures you are always prepared for new opportunities, specialty transitions, travel assignments, or leadership roles.

The Strategic Perspective

Think of your résumé not as a document that lists what you have done, but as a clinical readiness summary that answers an employer's key questions: Can this professional perform exams safely? Can they learn quickly? Will they communicate well with patients and physicians? Are they reliable enough to trust in a high-volume clinical environment? When your résumé clearly communicates those answers, interviews begin to follow.

A strong Diagnostic Medical Sonographer résumé is not flashy, complicated, or lengthy. It is clear, clinically focused, precise, and honest about competencies. When written well, it becomes more than a job application—it becomes the first signal that you are ready to step into the role with professionalism, discipline, and confidence.

Chapter 33

Behavioral Interviewing for Diagnostic Medical Sonographers

Why Healthcare Uses It — and How to Answer With Confidence

Many healthcare employers now rely heavily on **behavioral interviewing**, a structured method of interviewing based on one central assumption: past behavior is the best predictor of future performance. Rather than asking hypothetical questions such as "What would you do if...," hiring managers ask candidates to describe **real situations they have already handled**. This approach allows leaders to evaluate not only technical skill, but also judgment, communication style, emotional regulation, accountability, and teamwork—traits that directly affect patient safety and department culture.

In diagnostic medical sonography, behavioral interviewing is especially important because the role sits at the intersection of patient interaction, real-time clinical decision support, and workflow reliability. Employers want to understand how you behave when the schedule is overloaded, when a physician requests urgent additional images, when a patient becomes anxious, or when you recognize something unexpected during an exam. Technical ability can be taught; professional behavior under pressure is harder to change. Behavioral interviews help organizations identify candidates who are steady, coachable, and safe.

Why Healthcare Organizations Depend on Behavioral Interviewing

Healthcare environments are complex, fast-moving, and highly collaborative. Sonographers interact with radiologists, cardiologists, nurses, physicians, schedulers, and patients throughout every shift. Behavioral interviewing allows hiring leaders to evaluate whether a candidate communicates clearly, manages stress effectively, accepts feedback constructively, and maintains professionalism even in emotionally charged situations. Departments are not only hiring scanning ability; they are hiring reliability, teamwork, and patient-centered conduct.

Another reason behavioral interviewing is widely used is **consistency**. Structured behavioral questions allow interview panels to evaluate all candidates using the same criteria, which improves fairness and reduces hiring bias. For applicants, this means preparation becomes much easier once you understand the types of experiences employers want to hear about.

The STAR Method: Your Most Important Interview Tool

The most effective way to answer behavioral questions is the **STAR method**, which organizes responses into four parts:

- **Situation:** Briefly describe the setting or challenge.

• **Task:** Explain your responsibility in that moment.

• **Action:** Describe what you specifically did.

• **Result:** Share the outcome and what you learned.

Using this structure keeps answers focused and demonstrates clinical reasoning, not just storytelling.

Example structure:

"During my vascular clinical rotation (Situation), I was responsible for completing a lower-extremity venous Doppler exam on a patient with severe discomfort (Task). I explained each step slowly, adjusted positioning to reduce pain, and completed the protocol while communicating with the supervising technologist about possible limitations (Action). The exam was successfully completed without needing to reschedule, and I learned how small positioning adjustments can significantly improve patient tolerance (Result)."

Common Behavioral Interview Questions for Sonographers

Healthcare employers often ask variations of the following questions:

• Tell me about a time you handled a difficult patient.

• Describe a situation where you had to manage a high workload or time pressure.

• Tell me about a time you made a mistake and how you handled it.

• Describe a time you worked with a challenging team member.

- Tell me about a time you had to learn something quickly.
- Describe a situation where you identified a problem others did not notice.
- Tell me about a time you received critical feedback.

Preparing structured examples for these themes ensures you can respond calmly even if the wording changes.

Behavioral Interview Script Examples

1. Handling an Anxious Patient

"During my OB rotation, I scanned a patient who was visibly anxious because of a previous pregnancy complication. My responsibility was to complete the exam while helping the patient remain calm. I slowed my pace slightly, explained each step of the exam, and checked in periodically to ensure she was comfortable. By maintaining steady communication, the patient relaxed enough for the exam to be completed successfully, and the supervising sonographer later commented that the patient interaction improved exam quality. That experience reinforced the importance of balancing efficiency with emotional awareness."

2. Managing High Workload Pressure

"In my final clinical rotation, our department experienced an unusually high number of add-on ER studies during a single shift. I was responsible for assisting with abdominal exams while maintaining documentation accuracy. I organized my workflow by preparing supplies between patients, confirming exam priorities with the lead technologist, and double-checking labeling before finalizing images. Despite the high volume, we stayed on schedule and avoided repeat scans, which showed me how organization and communication help maintain quality even when pace increases."

3. Accepting Feedback and Improving Performance

"Early in my clinical training, a preceptor pointed out that I was taking longer than necessary to optimize images because I was over-adjusting settings. I asked for specific guidance, practiced recommended shortcuts, and reviewed images after each exam to monitor improvement. Within a few weeks, my scanning time improved significantly without sacrificing image quality. That experience taught me to treat feedback as a performance tool rather than criticism."

4. Identifying a Potential Issue During an Exam

"During a renal exam, I noticed a finding that seemed inconsistent with the patient's clinical history. Although I was still a student, I captured additional views and notified the supervising sonographer to review the images. The additional documentation helped ensure the interpreting physician had sufficient information. That situation reinforced the importance of documenting uncertainty carefully and communicating concerns early."

What Interviewers Are Really Listening For

When interviewers ask behavioral questions, they are not searching for perfect stories. They are evaluating how you think, how you communicate, and how you respond under pressure. Strong answers demonstrate accountability, collaboration, awareness of patient experience, willingness to ask for help, and commitment to learning. Even when discussing mistakes, the key is to show reflection and improvement rather than defensiveness.

Avoid vague responses such as “I always work well under pressure” or “I try my best with patients.” Instead, describe **specific situations** that illustrate how you behave in real clinical environments. Specificity builds credibility.

Preparing Before the Interview

Preparation does not require memorizing scripts. Instead, prepare five to seven short clinical stories that reflect common workplace situations: handling a challenging patient, managing workflow pressure, learning new equipment quickly, working through feedback, helping a teammate, or identifying a safety concern. Practice telling each story using the STAR structure so your responses feel natural rather than rehearsed. When you enter the interview with prepared examples, behavioral questions become much easier to answer confidently.

The Strategic Advantage

Behavioral interviewing can feel intimidating at first, but it actually benefits well-prepared candidates. Sonographers who demonstrate calm communication, reliability, humility, and patient-centered thinking often stand out even when competing against candidates with similar technical training. Departments want professionals who can be trusted not only to obtain accurate images, but also to represent the team professionally during difficult patient encounters and high-pressure situations.

The Bottom Line

Healthcare organizations use behavioral interviewing because clinical environments demand more than technical proficiency. They require judgment, composure, collaboration, and accountability. By preparing structured examples, practicing the STAR method, and reflecting on real clinical experiences, you can walk into interviews prepared to show not just what you know, but **how you work**. And in healthcare hiring, how you work often determines whether the offer follows.

Chapter 34

Interview and Job Search Guide for Sonographers

How to Find the Right Position, Impress Every Manager, and Start Your Career Strong

Introduction — You're Qualified. Now You Need to Be Strategic.

Graduation hits. Credentials arrive. Your badge feels shiny. Your hands feel ready. And then it hits you — you have to actually find a job. This chapter walks you through everything: résumés, cover letters, job boards, what managers look for, what red flags to avoid, how to talk about your skills, how to interview well, what to negotiate, and how to choose the right environment. By the end, readers will be able to walk into any interview with calm confidence and walk out with offers that actually fit their goals.

Part 1 — Finding the Right Jobs

Your first step matters more than you think. Start with the setting: hospital versus clinic. Hospitals typically offer higher pay, more specialties, stronger benefits, more call (which can mean both more income and more stress), faster growth opportunities, and exposure to trauma and emergencies. Clinics often provide predictable hours, lower emotional load, lower pay, no call requirements, and are often ideal for work-life balance. Choose based on your current season of life, not outside pressure.

Where to look for jobs includes hospital system websites, Indeed, LinkedIn, the SDMS Career Center, ARDMS job boards, radiology or vascular-specific boards, local healthcare Facebook groups, and word-of-mouth through clinical instructors. Most ultrasound jobs are never advertised publicly; many are filled through clinical rotations, networking, and internal referrals. Apply broadly but interview selectively. Apply to several hospitals, a few clinics, perhaps a travel agency or two if interested, and one or two dream jobs, then evaluate which align best with your life.

Part 2 — Crafting a Résumé That Actually Gets Interviews

Your résumé should be one page: clean, confident, and clear. Hiring managers skim, so readability matters. Include your name and credentials (RDMS, RVT, RDCS if applicable), contact information, clinical skills, scanning competencies, education and certifications, clinical rotation sites, technical abilities such as Doppler or elastography and specific machines, professional memberships, and optional volunteer work. Do not simply list tasks; list abilities. Instead of "Performed abdominal ultrasounds," write "Completed high-volume abdominal, pelvic, and OB exams; competent with Doppler analysis and pathology documentation." Managers want evidence of judgment, not just bullet points. Highlight what makes you employable immediately, such as proficiency across specialties, familiarity with systems like Epic or Cerner, strong patient communication skills, and the ability to perform STAT or ER exams.

Part 3 — The Cover Letter That Doesn't Sound Like a Template

A strong cover letter is short, warm, professional, specific, and confident without ego. Emphasize patient-centered care, eagerness to learn, teamwork, curiosity, and alignment with the department. Managers hire energy and sincerity, not long paragraphs.

Part 4 — What Hiring Managers Really Want

Reliability matters more than GPA. Managers look for candidates who are on time, prepared, and consistent. Trainability is equally important; they do not expect perfection, but they do expect coachability. Candidates who accept feedback with appreciation stand out immediately. Emotional self-control is essential because hospitals are chaotic environments where professionals must remain calm, respectful, and steady even under pressure. Compassion also matters deeply; professionals who remain kind during difficult scans are consistently valued.

Part 5 — Interview Preparation

Dress like a professional, not a student. Scrubs are often appropriate for hospital interviews, while business casual works well for clinics. Avoid wrinkled clothing, messy appearance, or visible stress signals. Bring a portfolio that includes your résumé, letters of recommendation, clinical evaluations, certifications, and a brief list of exams performed during training. Prepare to answer common questions confidently. When asked "Tell me about yourself," describe your path, your motivation for sonography, your specialty interests, and your clinical strengths. For "What is your biggest weakness?" choose something real but fixable, such as learning to slow down under pressure and double-checking images. When asked how you handle difficult patients, demonstrate empathy, boundaries, and calm communication. For "Why do you want to work here?" mention team culture, specialties, patient population, and alignment rather than generic compliments.

Part 6 — Questions You Must Ask Them

Asking thoughtful questions helps you avoid toxic environments. Ask about workflow, including the number of scans per day, whether support staff assist with room preparation, and whether you will handle most emergency exams. Ask about training, including whether you will have a dedicated preceptor and how long orientation lasts. Ask about equipment, including what machines are used and how frequently they are updated. Ask about call and overtime expectations because these directly affect income, schedule, sleep, and burnout risk.

Part 7 — Evaluating Red Flags

Be cautious of departments that say, "We don't really have an orientation," "We need someone fast," "You'll be fine — you'll figure it out," "We're always short-staffed," or "We don't have time for questions." These statements often signal weak leadership, burnout culture, or unsafe expectations.

Part 8 — Negotiating Your Offer

New graduates are often surprised to learn that polite negotiation is acceptable. You can ask about pay, shift differentials, call pay, sign-on bonuses, educational reimbursement, scrub allowances, PTO structure, and shift preferences. Confidence and professionalism matter more than aggressive negotiation tactics.

Part 9 — The First 90 Days

The first 90 days shape your reputation. Reliability is essential: never be late, always be prepared, and follow through on commitments. Take notes consistently by carrying a small notebook, recording anatomy landmarks, workflow tips, and scanning pearls. Ask for feedback weekly to demonstrate humility, accountability, and commitment to growth.

The Bottom Line

Getting hired as a Diagnostic Medical Sonographer is not just about technical skill; it is about professional presence. The individuals who receive offers are steady, curious, humble, teachable, compassionate, attentive, and reliable. This chapter provides the full playbook for approaching the job search with clarity, preparation, and confidence.

Chapter 35

The Never End

One day, long after your first nervous scans and your first carefully labeled images, you will realize something quietly powerful: this profession never truly ends. The machines evolve. The protocols update. New specialties emerge. New pathologies appear. Technology becomes faster, smarter, and more precise. Yet the core of the work remains beautifully unchanged — a trained set of hands, a disciplined eye, and a calm professional presence helping patients and clinicians see what cannot be seen any other way.

There will always be another anatomy variation to recognize, another technique to refine, another measurement to master, another patient who needs reassurance before the probe ever touches their skin. There will be days when the workflow feels heavy, when the department runs behind, and when your shoulders remind you that this work is physical as well as intellectual. And there will also be days when you catch something subtle that changes a patient's outcome, when a physician thanks you for your precision, or when a nervous patient relaxes simply because you spoke with steadiness and kindness. Those moments accumulate quietly into a career that matters more than most people outside healthcare ever fully realize.

Sonography is not a static skill you learn once and repeat forever. It is a lifelong practice. The professionals who thrive are not the ones who memorize the most protocols early; they are the ones who stay curious, stay teachable, protect their bodies, refine their judgment, and continue learning long after formal education ends. The field will continue to expand, and so will your role within it if you choose to keep growing alongside it.

So this is not the finish line of a book, and it is not the finish line of your training. It is the beginning of a professional journey that continues to unfold scan by scan, patient by patient, year by year. The learning does not end. The responsibility does not end. And the opportunity to make a meaningful difference — quietly, consistently, and skillfully — never ends.

Goodbye for now . . .

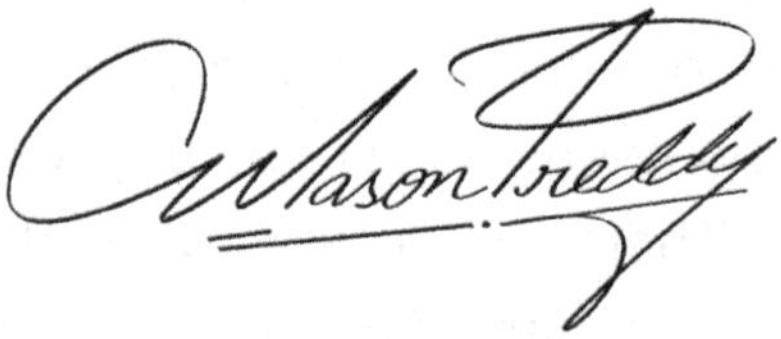

Chapter 36
About the Author

Mason Preddy has spent more than two and a half decades working at the intersection of healthcare recruitment, workforce strategy, retention, and career alignment. Throughout his career, he has partnered with hospitals, health systems, academic institutions, and national healthcare organizations to help clinicians not only find jobs, but find roles that match how they are wired, how they want to practice, and how they can sustain meaningful careers over time.

He is the creator of Mason's Alignment Theory (MAT), the **PACES™** and **CARESET™** alignment frameworks, and the *SCRUBfit™** Healthcare Career Assessment, tools designed to help current and future healthcare professionals understand the real daily demands of clinical roles before committing years of training, financial investment, and emotional energy. His work focuses on one central belief: burnout is not always a failure of resilience — it is often a failure of fit.

Mason is the founder of Mason Maison™ Publishing and the architect of the ScrubTales™ career guide series, a collection of real-world healthcare career books designed to move beyond job descriptions and reveal the lived realities, tradeoffs, and long-term pathways of healthcare professions. Through his writing, speaking, and workforce consulting, he continues to advocate for earlier career clarity, stronger retention through alignment, and more transparent conversations about what healthcare careers truly require.

Chapter 37

Also by Mason Maison™ Publishing

What Color Are Your Scrubs?

A comprehensive healthcare career guide exploring 345 healthcare professions through the lens of identity alignment, sustainability, and real-world career fit. Designed for students, career changers, and healthcare professionals seeking clarity before committing to long training pathways.

ScrubTales™ Career Guide Series

A growing series of real-world career guides that examine healthcare professions from the inside out—covering the daily realities of practice, long-term career sustainability, hiring pathways, financial tradeoffs, and the emotional and cognitive demands of each role.

Selected titles include:

ScrubTales™ Nurse Practitioner

A real-world career guide exploring clinical decision-making responsibility, specialty pathways, compensation structures, and long-term sustainability in advanced practice nursing.

ScrubTales™ Physician Assistant

An in-depth look at the versatility, specialty mobility, hiring dynamics, and long-term career flexibility of the physician assistant profession.

ScrubTales™ Registered Nurse

A practical exploration of nursing pathways, bedside realities, specialty transitions, and long-term career architecture across the nursing profession.

ScrubTales™ Surgical Technologist

A real-world guide to the operating room environment, surgical teamwork, sterile technique responsibilities, and the day-to-day realities of procedural care.

ScrubTales™ Diagnostic Medical Sonographer

A comprehensive career guide examining imaging specialties, technology evolution, hiring strategies, and the long-term professional trajectory of sonographers in modern healthcare.

Chapter 38

Glossary

Essential Terms for Diagnostic Medical Sonography

1. Acoustic Shadowing

A dark area on the ultrasound image where sound waves are blocked or absorbed, commonly seen behind stones or dense structures.

2. Acoustic Window

An area of the body that allows clear ultrasound penetration, used to visualize deeper organs.

3. Adenopathy

Enlargement of lymph nodes, often evaluated in oncology and general ultrasound.

4. Anechoic

A region that appears completely black on ultrasound because it reflects no sound waves, such as fluid-filled cysts.

5. Appendicitis

Inflammation of the appendix, often detected by identifying a non-compressible, enlarged tubular structure in the RLQ.

6. Artifact

An image distortion or false structure created by physics limitations or technical factors in ultrasound.

7. Ascites

Free fluid in the abdominal cavity.

8. Aseptic Technique

Practices used to prevent infection during procedures or scanning.

9. Attenuation

Loss of ultrasound wave strength as it travels through tissue.

10. Avascular

Lacking blood flow on Doppler evaluation.

11. Beam Steering

Adjusting the angle of the ultrasound beam without moving the transducer, used in vascular exams.

12. Bile Ducts

Tubes that carry bile from the liver and gallbladder to the intestine, commonly evaluated for obstruction.

13. Biopsy Guide

A device used to help direct a needle during ultrasound-guided procedures.

14. B-mode

Brightness mode imaging — the standard grayscale image used in ultrasound.

15. Calipers

Measurement markers used to assess size, length, depth, and diameter on ultrasound.

16. Cine Loop

A short video clip of ultrasound frames captured in sequence for review of moving anatomy.

17. Color Doppler

A technique that shows blood flow direction and velocity using color overlays.

18. Complex Mass

A structure containing both cystic (fluid) and solid components.

19. Compression Technique

Gentle pressure applied with the probe to assess compressibility of structures like veins or the appendix.

20. Cortex

The outer layer of an organ, such as the kidney or lymph node.

21. Cystic

Fluid-filled; usually appears anechoic with posterior enhancement.

22. Decubitus Position

A patient position lying on their side, often used for gallbladder and renal imaging.

23. Doppler Angle

The optimal angle (usually 45–60°) needed for accurate blood flow measurements.

24. Echogenic

Reflective on ultrasound — appears bright or white.

25. Echotexture

The pattern of echoes within tissue; used to assess normal vs abnormal appearance.

26. Effusion

Fluid collected in an anatomical space, such as the pleura or joint.

27. Elastography

Advanced ultrasound technique that measures tissue stiffness, often used in liver and oncology imaging.

28. Embolus

A clot or blockage traveling through the bloodstream.

29. Enlargement

Increase in size of an organ or structure; often evaluated in spleen, liver, kidneys, and lymph nodes.

30. Enhancement, Posterior

Increased brightness behind fluid-filled structures because sound waves pass easily through them.

31. FAST Exam

Focused Assessment with Sonography in Trauma; a rapid bedside scan to detect internal bleeding.

32. Fetal Biometry

Measurements taken during an obstetric exam to assess fetal growth.

33. Fetal Heart Rate

The baby's heartbeat measured during OB ultrasound; typically between 110–160 bpm.

34. Fibroid

A benign tumor of the uterus that appears solid and well-circumscribed on ultrasound.

35. Flow Reversal

Abnormal blood flow direction seen on Doppler, often indicating severe vascular disease.

36. Gaiting

Using ECG signals during cardiac ultrasound to time image acquisition with the cardiac cycle.

37. Gain

A setting that adjusts the brightness of the ultrasound image.

38. Gestational Sac

The first visible structure of early pregnancy seen on ultrasound.

39. Grayscale Imaging

Standard black-and-white ultrasound that shows tissue structure and density.

40. Hemangioma

A benign liver lesion with characteristic hyperechoic appearance.

41. Hematoma

A collection of blood in soft tissue, often appearing complex or heterogeneous.

42. Hemodynamics

The study of blood flow and pressure, important in vascular ultrasound.

43. Hepatomegaly

Enlargement of the liver.

44. Hilum

The central part of an organ where vessels and ducts enter and exit, such as in the kidney or lymph node.

45. Heterogeneous

Tissue that appears mixed or uneven on ultrasound.

46. Homogeneous

Tissue with a uniform texture and appearance.

47. Hydronephrosis

Dilation of the kidney's collecting system, usually from obstruction.

48. Hyperechoic

Brighter than surrounding tissue; reflects many sound waves.

49. Hypoechoic

Darker than surrounding tissue; reflects fewer sound waves.

50. IVC (Inferior Vena Cava)

A large abdominal vein returning blood to the heart; often evaluated for thrombus or volume status.

51. Image Optimization

Adjusting settings like depth, gain, and focus to improve clarity.

52. Isoechoic

Having the same brightness as surrounding tissues.

53. Jugular Vein

A major neck vein assessed during vascular ultrasound.

54. Kidney Cortex

The outer part of the kidney where filtration occurs; echogenicity can reveal disease.

55. Ligamentum Teres

A fibrous remnant in the liver used as a landmark during abdominal scanning.

56. Longitudinal View

An imaging plane showing the structure lengthwise.

57. Lymph Node

A small immune structure often evaluated for enlargement, shape, or abnormal internal architecture.

58. M-Mode

Motion mode used to measure movement, commonly in cardiac and fetal heart exams.

59. Mass Effect

Pressure from a mass that displaces or distorts nearby anatomy.

60. Murphy's Sign (Ultrasound)

Pain when the sonographer presses over the gallbladder, indicating inflammation.

61. Necrosis

Death of tissue, often appearing as irregular, avascular, or heterogeneous areas on ultrasound.

62. Neonatal Head Ultrasound

A scan performed through the fontanelle of a newborn to evaluate the brain for bleeds or abnormalities.

63. NPO

A patient instruction meaning "nothing by mouth" before certain abdominal exams.

64. Obstruction

Blockage of ducts, vessels, or organs that disrupts normal flow, often diagnosed via ultrasound.

65. Ovarian Cyst

A fluid-filled structure in the ovary; commonly simple, complex, or hemorrhagic.

66. Pancreatitis

Inflammation of the pancreas, often showing hypoechoic enlargement and peripancreatic fluid.

67. Parasternal View

A standard cardiac imaging window used to visualize the heart in long and short axis.

68. Parenchyma

The functional tissue of an organ, such as liver or kidney, evaluated for texture and disease.

69. Pelvic Free Fluid

Fluid within the pelvis, often visualized in the cul-de-sac or adnexal regions.

70. Pericardial Effusion

Fluid around the heart.

71. Peristalsis

Movement of bowel loops; lack of peristalsis may indicate obstruction or inflammation.

72. Plaque (Vascular)

A buildup of fatty or calcified material inside arteries, evaluated during Doppler studies.

73. Pleural Effusion

Fluid in the chest cavity surrounding the lungs.

74. Portal Vein

A major vein bringing blood from the intestines to the liver; assessed for flow, thrombus, or portal hypertension.

75. Portosystemic Flow

Abnormal flow patterns in the liver caused by portal hypertension or shunting.

76. Posterior Enhancement

Increased brightness behind fluid-filled structures, aiding in diagnosis of cysts.

77. Probe Marker

The physical indicator on a transducer that aligns with orientation markers on the screen.

78. Pseudocyst

A fluid collection, often in the pancreas, lacking epithelial lining.

79. Pulmonary Hypertension

High pressure in the pulmonary arteries, sometimes inferred during echocardiography.

80. Pyloric Stenosis

A condition in infants where the pylorus thickens, diagnosed with specific ultrasound measurements.

81. Radiologist

A physician specializing in interpreting medical imaging studies, including ultrasound.

82. Real-Time Imaging

The ability of ultrasound to show moving anatomy, such as blood flow or fetal movement.

83. Renal Artery Stenosis

Narrowing of the renal arteries, evaluated through Doppler for peak velocities and waveform changes.

84. Resistive Index (RI)

A Doppler measurement evaluating vascular resistance, especially in kidneys.

85. Reversal of Flow

Abnormal backward blood flow, often indicating severe disease.

86. Reverberation Artifact

Repeating bands or echoes caused by sound bouncing between structures.

87. Right Upper Quadrant (RUQ)

An abdominal region containing the liver, gallbladder, and right kidney.

88. Sagittal Plane

An imaging plane dividing the body into right and left sections.

89. Septations

Thin internal walls within a cyst or fluid collection.

90. Shadowing

An artifact where a strong reflector blocks sound waves, creating a dark region behind it.

91. Side Lobe Artifact

Unwanted echoes produced by off-axis ultrasound beams, creating false structures.

92. Simple Cyst

A fluid-filled structure with smooth walls, anechoic center, and posterior enhancement.

93. Sonographer

A trained healthcare professional who performs diagnostic ultrasound examinations.

94. Spectral Doppler

A Doppler display that shows blood flow velocity over time in waveform form.

95. Splenomegaly

Enlargement of the spleen, commonly assessed during abdominal ultrasound.

96. Stenosis

Narrowing of a vessel or duct, often identified by elevated Doppler velocities.

97. Subcutaneous Tissue

The layer of fat and connective tissue beneath the skin.

98. Subhepatic Space

The area beneath the liver where fluid can collect.

99. Suprarenal

Located above the kidneys, often referring to the adrenal glands.

100. Tachycardia

A heart rate above the normal range, often visible on M-mode or Doppler.

101. Target Sign

A specific sonographic pattern resembling concentric rings, commonly seen in intussusception.

102. Thrombus

A blood clot within a vessel, appearing echogenic or heterogeneous depending on age.

103. Thyroid Isthmus

The thin band of thyroid tissue connecting the right and left lobes.

104. Torsion

Twisting of an organ, such as an ovary or testicle, causing loss of blood flow.

105. Transducer

The handheld device that generates and receives ultrasound waves.

106. Transverse Plane

An imaging plane that divides the body into superior and inferior portions.

107. Triphasic Flow

A normal arterial Doppler waveform with forward, reverse, and forward components.

108. Tumor Margins

The edges of a mass, assessed for smoothness or irregularity.

109. Ultrasound Contrast

Microbubble agents used to enhance vascular imaging, especially in cardiac and liver exams.

110. Ultrasonography

The medical use of high-frequency sound waves to create real-time images of internal structures.

111. Umbilical Artery Doppler

A fetal Doppler assessment used to evaluate placental blood flow.

112. Unilateral

Affecting one side of the body or organ system.

113. Valsalva Maneuver

A breathing technique used during vascular exams to assess venous function.

114. Varicocele

Dilated veins in the scrotum, often showing increased size with Valsalva.

115. Vascular Resistance

Opposition to blood flow within vessels, assessed using Doppler indices.

116. Venous Insufficiency

Poor venous valve function causing reflux, identified on Doppler.

117. Ventricular Hypertrophy

Thickening of the heart's ventricular walls, evaluated during cardiac ultrasound.

118. Waveform Analysis

Interpreting the shape, peaks, and patterns of Doppler tracings to assess vascular health.

119. Whirl Sign

A twisted appearance of vessels or structures, often seen in cases of torsion.

120. Window (Acoustic)

An anatomical area that allows optimal visualization of deeper structures.

121. Acoustic Impedance

The resistance a material offers to the passage of sound waves, affecting how echoes appear on ultrasound.

122. Alveoli

Tiny air sacs in the lungs that cause strong shadowing because ultrasound cannot pass through air.

123. Aneuploidy Markers

Ultrasound findings that may indicate chromosomal abnormalities during pregnancy.

124. Annular Pancreas

A congenital condition where pancreatic tissue encircles the duodenum, sometimes seen in abdominal scans.

125. Aortomesenteric Angle

The angle between the aorta and superior mesenteric artery, assessed in suspected SMA syndrome.

126. Apical View

A cardiac imaging window obtained from the chest apex to visualize chambers and valves.

127. Ascending Aorta

The upward section of the aorta emerging from the heart, evaluated in cardiac ultrasound.

128. Atrophy

Decrease in size of an organ or tissue, often appearing hyperechoic or shrunken.

129. Bicornuate Uterus

A congenital uterine anomaly with two horn-like cavities.

130. B-lines

Vertical reverberation artifacts seen in lung ultrasound that may indicate pulmonary edema.

131. Calyces

Cup-shaped structures within the kidneys that collect urine.

132. Carotid Bulb

The widened portion of the carotid artery prone to plaque formation.

133. Cavernous Transformation

Multiple small veins developing around a chronically blocked portal vein.

134. Choledocholithiasis

Gallstones lodged in the common bile duct.

135. Chorionicity

Refers to whether twins share the same placental structures.

136. Clot Burden

The extent or amount of thrombus present in a vessel.

137. Collagenous Tissue

Connective tissue that can appear hyperechoic on ultrasound.

138. Complex Fluid

Fluid containing debris, septations, or internal echoes, suggesting infection or hemorrhage.

139. Congenital Anomaly

A structural abnormality present at birth, often detected during prenatal ultrasound.

140. Contour

The shape or outline of an organ or lesion, used to assess pathology.

141. Cul-de-sac

The space behind the uterus where pelvic free fluid often accumulates.

142. Decidual Reaction

A thickened uterine lining seen in early pregnancy.

143. Dicrotic Notch

A small dip in arterial waveforms representing aortic valve closure.

144. Diastole

The phase of the cardiac cycle when the heart relaxes and fills with blood.

145. Dilatation

Widening or stretching of a structure, such as a duct or vessel.

146. Doppler Shift

The change in frequency of returning sound waves used to calculate blood flow velocity.

147. Duplex Ultrasound

Combines grayscale imaging with spectral Doppler to assess vessels.

148. Echogenic Foci

Small bright spots within organs, sometimes normal and sometimes pathological.

149. Ectopic Pregnancy

A pregnancy located outside the uterus, often in the fallopian tube.

150. Edema

Swelling caused by excess fluid in tissues, often appearing hypoechoic.

151. Effacement

Thinning of the cervix during pregnancy, sometimes evaluated on transvaginal ultrasound.

152. Embryo

The early stage of human development before becoming a fetus.

153. Endometrium

The inner lining of the uterus, evaluated for thickness, texture, and phases.

154. Endometrioma

A type of ovarian cyst filled with old blood, often appearing homogeneous and low-level echogenic.

155. Enlargement Ratio

A measurement comparing organ sizes to normal ranges to evaluate pathology.

156. Enthesitis

Inflammation at tendon attachment sites, sometimes seen in musculoskeletal ultrasound.

157. Epigastric Region

Upper central abdominal area containing the stomach and pancreas.

158. Epithelium

The tissue lining organs and cavities, sometimes identified in cyst wall assessments.

159. Ergonomics

Proper body positioning during scanning to prevent musculoskeletal injury.

160. Extratesticular Mass

A mass located outside the testicle, often benign.

161. Falx Cerebri

A midline structure in the brain used as a landmark in neonatal head ultrasound.

162. Femoral Vein

A major vein in the leg assessed for thrombus during vascular ultrasound.

163. Fetal Pole

The first visible sign of an embryo on early pregnancy ultrasound.

164. Fetal Presentation

The part of the fetus closest to the cervix, such as cephalic or breech.

165. Fibrosis

Thickening or scarring of tissue, often causing increased echogenicity.

166. Flow Phasicity

The natural variation of venous or arterial flow during respiration or heartbeat.

167. Fontanelle

Soft spots in an infant's skull used as acoustic windows for head ultrasound.

168. Foramen Ovale

A fetal heart structure that allows blood flow between atria before birth.

169. Fusiform Aneurysm

A spindle-shaped dilation of a vessel.

170. Gallbladder Sludge

Thickened bile that appears as low-level echoes without shadowing.

171. Gas Artifact

Distortion caused by air in the bowel or stomach, blocking sound waves.

172. Gestational Age

The age of a pregnancy calculated from the last menstrual period.

173. GFR (Glomerular Filtration Rate)

A measure of kidney function sometimes correlated with sonographic findings.

174. HCG (Human Chorionic Gonadotropin)

A hormone used to correlate early pregnancy ultrasound findings.

175. Heel-Toe Maneuver

A probe technique used to fine-tune angles and improve visualization.

176. Hepatopedal Flow

Portal vein blood flow moving toward the liver, the normal direction.

177. Hepatofugal Flow

Portal vein blood flow moving away from the liver, often indicating severe disease.

178. Hilum Flow Pattern

Normal vascular flow seen entering organs like lymph nodes or kidneys.

179. Homograft

A transplanted tissue from a donor of the same species, sometimes assessed with ultrasound.

180. Hydrocele

Fluid surrounding the testicle, appearing anechoic on ultrasound.

181. Hydrosalpinx

A fluid-filled fallopian tube, typically appearing tubular and anechoic or with incomplete septations.

182. Hyperemia

Increased blood flow on Doppler, often indicating inflammation or infection.

183. Hypoplastic

Underdeveloped tissue or organ, often identified during pediatric or fetal ultrasound.

184. Iliac Arteries

Major pelvic arteries visualized during abdominal and vascular studies.

185. Iliac Veins

Large veins in the pelvis evaluated during DVT studies.

186. Inferior Pole

The lower portion of an organ, often referenced in kidney scanning.

187. Infertility Evaluation

Ultrasound assessment for causes of infertility, including ovarian reserve and uterine structure.

188. Inguinal Region

The groin area where hernias and lymph nodes are frequently evaluated.

189. Inhomogeneous

Another term for heterogeneous—mixed echogenicity within tissue.

190. Inlet Flow

Blood entering a chamber, vessel, or graft, evaluated by Doppler.

191. Interlobar Arteries

Renal arteries located between the kidney pyramids used for RI measurements.

192. Intima-Media Thickness (IMT)

A vascular measurement used to assess atherosclerosis.

193. Intussusception

A pediatric condition where bowel telescopes into itself, showing the characteristic “target sign.”

194. Invasive Procedure

A medical procedure involving entry into the body, sometimes assisted by ultrasound guidance.

195. Inversion Mode

An imaging technique emphasizing fluid-filled structures, often used in obstetrics.

196. Ischemia

Reduced blood flow causing tissue damage, often evaluated via Doppler patterns.

197. Isthmus

A thin connecting tissue band, commonly referring to the thyroid isthmus.

198. Jugular Reflux

Backward flow in the jugular vein during certain maneuvers, assessed during venous studies.

199. Kidney Pelvis

The central collecting area of the kidney where urine collects before entering the ureter.

200. KUB Region

An abbreviation for kidneys, ureters, and bladder — common in abdominal ultrasound.

201. Laminar Flow

Smooth, orderly blood flow seen as a clean, narrow Doppler spectrum.

202. Ligament of Treitz

An anatomical landmark separating the upper and lower GI tract, sometimes referenced in abdominal scans.

203. Linear Transducer

A high-frequency ultrasound probe used for superficial structures and vascular studies.

204. Liver Parenchyma

The functional tissue of the liver, evaluated for echotexture and disease.

205. Lobulated Margin

An irregular or scalloped edge of a lesion, sometimes concerning for malignancy.

206. Long-Axis View

An imaging plane that shows the full length of a structure.

207. Lumen

The inner space of a vessel or tubular structure.

208. Lymphadenopathy

Disease or enlargement of lymph nodes.

209. Macrosomia

A condition where a fetus has an unusually large size, assessed via biometry.

210. Main Portal Vein

The central vessel supplying the liver, routinely evaluated for size, flow direction, and thrombus.

Chapter 39

Bonus Glossary

Essential Terms for Diagnostic Medical Sonography — Intro

Diagnostic medical sonography is a profession with its own language, and it's not optional. The terms in this glossary are the words you will hear in exam rooms, read in orders, see in protocols, and use when you document studies that physicians will interpret and patients will depend on. Some of these terms describe ultrasound physics and image behavior, others describe anatomy and pathology, and many describe the decisions that separate a routine scan from a clinically meaningful exam. Learning this vocabulary early reduces cognitive load, improves confidence during scanning, and makes communication cleaner with radiologists, cardiologists, vascular teams, OB providers, and the colleagues who will train you, correct you, and eventually trust you.

Use this glossary as a working tool, not a one-time read. Skim it before clinical days. Revisit it when a preceptor drops a term you haven't heard before. Look up words immediately after a difficult exam so you can attach meaning to a real patient case, because that is how memory sticks. Over time, these terms stop feeling like definitions and start feeling like instinct, which is exactly the point. Sonography is part art, part science, and part disciplined repetition, and your language has to grow alongside your hands.

Bonus! 100 Additional Words Every Diagnostic Medical Sonographer Should Begin Learning

The essential glossary builds your foundation, but real sonography life moves fast, and the vocabulary expands quickly once you step into specialties. In practice, you will hear shorthand from emergency clinicians during FAST exams, nuanced measurement language in OB, waveform vocabulary in vascular, window and view language in echo, and procedural phrasing when ultrasound becomes the tool guiding real-time interventions. This bonus list is designed to accelerate that next layer of fluency. These are the kinds of words that show up in handoffs, in radiology conversations, in chart notes, and in the quick "can you take a look at this?" moments that shape your reputation.

Treat this list like a personal curriculum. Pick ten words at a time. Look them up, then listen for them on shift. Write them down after you hear them used in context, because context turns vocabulary into competence. The goal is not to sound impressive; the goal is to understand what your team is asking, recognize what matters in the scan, and communicate clearly when something is urgent, uncertain, or needs another set of eyes. The more fluent you become, the safer you become, and in sonography, safety is the quiet superpower that lasts an entire career.

1. Acoustic Enhancement

Acoustic enhancement — Increased echo brightness deep to fluid-filled structures because sound waves pass through fluid with minimal attenuation.

2. Aliasing

Aliasing — A Doppler artifact that occurs when blood flow velocity exceeds the Nyquist limit, causing incorrect color or spectral display.

3. Angle Correction

Angle correction — Adjustment of the Doppler cursor to align with blood flow direction to ensure accurate velocity measurement.

4. Aortic Root

Aortic root — The proximal portion of the aorta emerging from the heart, commonly measured in cardiac ultrasound.

5. Apical Four-Chamber View

Apical four-chamber view — A cardiac imaging window displaying both atria and ventricles simultaneously for structural and functional assessment.

6. Artifact Reduction

Artifact reduction — Techniques used to minimize image distortions caused by physics limitations or improper machine settings.

7. Baseline Shift

Baseline shift — Adjustment of the Doppler waveform baseline to better visualize high-velocity flow without truncation.

8. Beam Focusing

Beam focusing — Narrowing the ultrasound beam at a specific depth to improve lateral resolution.

9. Bowel Gas

Bowel gas — Air within the intestines that reflects ultrasound waves and may obscure deeper structures.

10. Cardiac Output

Cardiac output — The volume of blood pumped by the heart per minute, sometimes estimated using echocardiographic measurements.

11. Carotid Intima

Carotid intima — The inner layer of the carotid artery wall evaluated when assessing vascular disease.

12. Cavitation

Cavitation — Formation of microscopic gas bubbles in tissue due to ultrasound pressure changes, typically minimal in diagnostic imaging.

13. Cephalic Presentation

Cephalic presentation — Fetal position in which the head is oriented toward the birth canal.

14. Collateral Circulation

Collateral circulation — Alternative blood flow pathways that develop when primary vessels are obstructed.

15. Contrast Harmonic Imaging

Contrast harmonic imaging — Ultrasound technique using contrast agents and harmonic signals to enhance vascular visualization.

16. Continuous Wave Doppler

Continuous wave Doppler — Doppler method that continuously transmits and receives signals to measure very high velocities without depth specificity.

17. Cord Doppler

Cord Doppler — Doppler evaluation of blood flow within the umbilical cord vessels.

18. Critical Velocity

Critical velocity — A blood flow velocity threshold suggesting significant vessel narrowing.

19. Cross-Sectional Area

Cross-sectional area — The measured internal area of a vessel or structure, used in flow calculations.

20. Diastolic Flow

Diastolic flow — Blood movement occurring during the relaxation phase of the cardiac cycle.

21. Doppler Gate

Doppler gate — The selected sample volume from which Doppler signals are obtained.

22. Doppler Scale

Doppler scale — Velocity range displayed on the Doppler screen determining sensitivity to flow speed.

23. Dynamic Range

Dynamic range — The range of echo intensities displayed, influencing image contrast.

24. Echogenicity Comparison

Echogenicity comparison — Evaluation of tissue brightness relative to surrounding structures.

25. End-Diastolic Velocity

End-diastolic velocity — Blood flow velocity measured at the end of the heart's relaxation phase.

26. End-Systolic Velocity

End-systolic velocity — Velocity measurement obtained at the end of cardiac contraction.

27. Envelope Tracing

Envelope tracing — Manual or automatic outlining of the Doppler waveform to calculate velocity indices.

28. Fetal Lie

Fetal lie — Orientation of the fetus relative to the maternal spine (longitudinal, transverse, or oblique).

29. Flow Turbulence

Flow turbulence — Chaotic blood flow pattern often occurring near stenotic regions.

30. Focal Zone

Focal zone — The region of best image resolution at the depth where the beam is focused.

31. Gallbladder Wall Thickening

Gallbladder wall thickening — Increase in gallbladder wall measurement, often associated with inflammation or systemic disease.

32. Harmonic Imaging

Harmonic imaging — Technique that uses harmonic frequencies to improve image clarity and reduce artifacts.

33. Hemoperitoneum

Hemoperitoneum — Blood within the peritoneal cavity detected on ultrasound.

34. Hepatic Vein Waveform

Hepatic vein waveform — Doppler flow pattern reflecting right atrial pressure changes.

35. High-Frequency Probe

High-frequency probe — Transducer providing superior resolution for superficial structures but limited depth penetration.

36. Image Persistence

Image persistence — Retention of previous frames to smooth motion on the display.

37. Inferior Vena Cava Collapsibility

Inferior vena cava collapsibility — Measurement of IVC diameter changes during respiration to estimate volume status.

38. Intercostal Window

Intercostal window — Imaging approach between the ribs to visualize thoracic or upper abdominal structures.

39. Lateral Resolution

Lateral resolution — Ability to distinguish two structures positioned side-by-side.

40. Left Ventricular Ejection Fraction

Left ventricular ejection fraction — Percentage of blood ejected from the left ventricle with each contraction.

41. Linear Array

Linear array — Transducer producing a rectangular image commonly used for vascular and superficial imaging.

42. Low-Resistance Flow

Low-resistance flow — Doppler pattern characterized by continuous forward flow throughout the cardiac cycle.

43. Mechanical Index

Mechanical index — Indicator of ultrasound output related to the likelihood of cavitation.

44. Mesenteric Flow

Mesenteric flow — Blood circulation within intestinal vessels evaluated in vascular studies.

45. Mirror Artifact

Mirror artifact — Duplication of structures caused by reflection from a strong interface.

46. Motion Artifact

Motion artifact — Image distortion resulting from patient or probe movement.

47. Multiplanar Imaging

Multiplanar imaging — Visualization of structures in multiple scanning planes for comprehensive assessment.

48. Near Field

Near field — The region closest to the transducer where beam convergence begins.

49. Noncompressible Vein

Noncompressible vein — A vein that does not collapse with probe pressure, suggesting thrombosis.

50. Nyquist Limit

Nyquist limit — Maximum measurable Doppler velocity before aliasing occurs.

51. Organomegaly

Organomegaly — Enlargement of an organ beyond normal size.

52. Outflow Tract

Outflow tract — Pathway through which blood exits the heart ventricles.

53. Paradoxical Motion

Paradoxical motion — Abnormal movement of cardiac structures opposite expected direction.

54. Peak Systolic Velocity

Peak systolic velocity — Highest blood flow velocity during cardiac contraction.

55. Penetration Depth

Penetration depth — Maximum imaging depth achievable with adequate signal strength.

56. Perinephric Fluid

Perinephric fluid — Fluid collection surrounding the kidney.

57. Peripheral Resistance

Peripheral resistance — Opposition to blood flow within distal vascular beds.

58. Phased Array

Phased array — Transducer type using electronic steering to create sector-shaped images.

59. Portal Hypertension

Portal hypertension — Elevated pressure within the portal venous system.

60. Power Doppler

Power Doppler — Doppler technique displaying flow strength rather than direction.

61. Pulsatility Index

Pulsatility index — Doppler calculation reflecting resistance to blood flow.

62. Pulsed Wave Doppler

Pulsed wave Doppler — Doppler method measuring velocities at a specific depth.

63. Range Ambiguity

Range ambiguity — Inability to determine precise depth of returning echoes when pulse timing overlaps.

64. Rayleigh Scattering

Rayleigh scattering — Reflection of sound waves by structures smaller than the wavelength.

65. Recanalization

Recanalization — Reopening of a previously occluded vessel.

66. Reflector Interface

Reflector interface — Boundary between tissues where ultrasound waves reflect.

67. Renal Collecting System

Renal collecting system — Kidney structures that channel urine toward the ureter.

68. Resolution Tradeoff

Resolution tradeoff — Balance between penetration and image clarity when adjusting frequency.

69. Retrograde Flow

Retrograde flow — Blood moving opposite the normal direction.

70. Reverberation Reduction

Reverberation reduction — Techniques to minimize repeated echo artifacts.

71. Sampling Volume

Sampling volume — Region within the Doppler gate where flow is measured.

72. Scan Plane Adjustment

Scan plane adjustment — Altering probe orientation to improve visualization.

73. Sector Scan

Sector scan — Wedge-shaped imaging format produced by phased array transducers.

74. Septal Motion

Septal motion — Movement of the heart's interventricular septum during contraction.

75. Signal-to-Noise Ratio

Signal-to-noise ratio — Relationship between useful echo information and background interference.

76. Slice Thickness Artifact

Slice thickness artifact — False echoes created by structures outside the primary imaging plane.

77. Soft Tissue Interface

Soft tissue interface — Boundary between different soft tissues producing echoes.

78. Spatial Resolution

Spatial resolution — Ability to distinguish two separate structures in the image.

79. Spectral Broadening

Spectral broadening — Widening of Doppler waveform indicating turbulent flow.

80. Speckle Reduction

Speckle reduction — Image processing technique that smooths granular noise.

81. Standing Waves

Standing waves — Artifact produced by repeated reflections between two interfaces.

82. Static Image Capture

Static image capture — Freezing a single ultrasound frame for measurement or documentation.

83. Subcostal View

Subcostal view — Imaging approach beneath the rib cage commonly used in cardiac scanning.

84. Systolic Upstroke

Systolic upstroke — Initial rise of the Doppler waveform during cardiac contraction.

85. Temporal Resolution

Temporal resolution — Ability to accurately display rapid motion over time.

86. Tissue Harmonics

Tissue harmonics — Harmonic frequencies generated by tissue interaction that improve image clarity.

87. Tissue Interface

Tissue interface — Boundary between different tissues affecting reflection patterns.

88. Time Gain Compensation

Time gain compensation — Depth-based gain adjustment used to equalize image brightness.

89. Transducer Footprint

Transducer footprint — Contact surface area of the ultrasound probe.

90. Triphasic Waveform Loss

Triphasic waveform loss — Transition from normal triphasic arterial flow to biphasic or monophasic patterns indicating disease.

91. Turbulent Flow Pattern

Turbulent flow pattern — Irregular Doppler waveform indicating disturbed blood flow.

92. Ultrasound Beam Width

Ultrasound beam width — Thickness of the sound beam affecting image resolution.

93. Velocity Ratio

Velocity ratio — Comparison of blood flow velocities used to assess stenosis severity.

94. Vessel Patency

Vessel patency — Condition of a vessel remaining open and unobstructed.

95. Wall Filter

Wall filter — Doppler setting removing low-frequency signals from vessel wall motion.

96. Wave Reflection

Wave reflection — Return of ultrasound waves after striking tissue interfaces.

97. Window Optimization

Window optimization — Adjusting scanning approach to obtain the clearest acoustic window.

98. Workflow Protocol

Workflow protocol — Standardized sequence of scanning steps used for consistent exams.

99. Zero Flow Baseline

Zero flow baseline — Reference line on Doppler display representing no movement.

100. Zonal Imaging

Zonal imaging — Technique that uses multiple focal zones to improve image clarity across depths.

Chapter 40

Made in the USA
Monee, IL
05 November 2026

67911911R00177